Psychology for Midwives

Pregnancy, Childbirth and Puerperium

Psychology for Midwives

Pregnancy, Childbirth and Puerperium

Maureen Raynor and Carole England

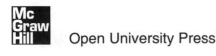
Open University Press

Open University Press
McGraw-Hill Education
McGraw-Hill House
Shoppenhangers Road
Maidenhead
Berkshire
England
SL6 2QL

email: enquiries@openup.co.uk
world wide web: www.openup.co.uk

and Two Penn Plaza, New York, NY 10121-2289, USA

First published 2010

A catalogue record of this book is available from the British Library

ISBN-13: 978-0-33-523433-2 (pb) 978-0-33-523432-5 (hb)
ISBN-10: 033523433X (pb) 0335234321 (hb)

Library of Congress Cataloging-in-Publication Data
CIP data applied for

Typeset by RefineCatch Limited, Bungay, Suffolk
Printed in the UK by Bell and Bain Ltd, Glasgow

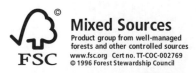

Mixed Sources
Product group from well-managed
forests and other controlled sources
www.fsc.org Cert no. TT-COC-002769
© 1996 Forest Stewardship Council

The McGraw·Hill Companies

In loving memory of both our fathers

Praise for *Psychology for Midwives* by Maureen Raynor and Carole England

"This is a lucid, well referenced and up-to-date text that will reward both the student and the practitioner . . . It is accessible and easy to read with numerous practical examples throughout the text . . . Chapter topics cover all the important areas but above all, in a profession whose effectiveness is arguably mediated primarily through relationships, the authors update all of us on the therapeutic nuances of these. This should definitely be your Psychology book of choice for the coming years. Read and enjoy . . ."

Dr Denis Walsh, Associate Professor in Midwifery, University of Nottingham, UK

Contents

About the authors   xi

Acknowledgements   xiii

Introduction   xv

1   Theoretical approaches to psychology and their
application to midwifery practice   1

Introduction
Chapter aims
The major approaches to
   psychology
Psychologies that have evolved
   the five major approaches
Alternative approaches to
   psychology

Conclusion
Summary of key points
References
Annotated further reading
Useful website

2   The mother–midwife relationship   15

Introduction
Chapter aims
Being with woman: establishing
   and building relationships
Constraining factors

Significant others
Conclusion
Summary of key points
References
Annotated further reading

3   Emotions during pregnancy, labour and puerperium   29

Introduction
Chapter aims
The link between the social
   and psychological dimensions
   of pregnancy, labour and
   the puerperium
Transitional crises
Motherhood
Fatherhood

Normative adjustment reactions
   during pregnancy, labour
   and the puerperium
Conclusion
Summary of key points
References
Annotated further reading
Useful websites

4   Perinatal mental illness   51

Introduction
Chapter aims
Clarification of terms
Why maternal mental health
   matters

Screening for mental illness:
   prediction and detection
Screening tools
Perinatal psychiatry
   disorders

Antenatal period – psychiatric
    disorders in pregnancy
Types of disorder in pregnancy
Serious mental illnesses
Postnatal period: serious
    psychiatric conditions
Mother–baby relationship
Care/management
Postnatal depressive illnesses
Mother–baby relationship
Care/management
Mild postpartum mood disorders
Mild postnatal depressive illness

Relationship with partner
Role of the midwife: learning
    lessons from key reports
Managed care networks
Suicide
Medical conditions caused by or
    mistaken for psychiatric disorder
Sharing best practice
Conclusion
Summary of key points
References
Annotated further reading
Useful websites

5   The psychology of communication in midwifery
    practice   82

Introduction
Chapter aims
The psychology of communication:
    the holistic approach
Building the working alliance:
    the rapport
The psychology of the first
    impression
Beyond first impressions:
    the psychology of building a
    relationship
Qualities of the midwife as an
    effective communicator
Relating in depth with other
    people – does it happen?

Assertiveness: the key to successful
    communication
The humanistic approach to
    communication
Listening and attending: the essential
    communication skills for
    woman-centred care
Listening, presence and touch
Barriers, constraints and difficulties
    that influence effective
    communication
Conclusion
Summary of key points
References
Annotated further reading

6   The birth environment   102

Introduction
Chapter aims
Critical appraisal of the evidence
Emotional work
Perception of pain:
    psychological factors

Conclusion
Summary of key points
References
Annotated further reading
Useful websites

7   The psychology of stress, anxiety and coping   121

Introduction
Chapter aims
Psychology of the self:
    self-knowledge
Defending the self from stresses
    and inconsistencies
The relationship between stress
    and coping

Coping strategies and midwifery
    practice
The related states of fear, anxiety,
    stress and emotion
Self-efficacy and coping
Control and coping
Fear, anxiety and birthing, not a
    winning combination

Conclusion   Annotated further reading
Summary of key points   Website
References

8   Psychosocial support   143
Introduction   Models of good practice
Chapter aims   Role of the midwife
What is psychosocial support?   Conclusion
Dimensions of support   Summary of key points
What does the evidence say?   References
Continuity of carer: is it important   Annotated further reading
  to women?   Useful websites
Type of care giver – who should
  support women during labour?

9   Attachment and bonding: the midwife's role in
     supporting parent–baby relationships   156
Introduction   Postnatal activities commonly
Chapter aims   associated with maternal
Development of the fetal mind   bonding/relationship building
  in preparation for emotional   When separation of parents and baby
  interactive relationships   is needed
Is the baby primed to attach?   Case study: Julie
Is the mother primed to make an   Case study: Lara
  affectionate bond to her baby?   So what can the midwife do?
Meeting their baby for the first   Conclusion
  time   Summary of key points
Mother and baby communication   References
  mediated through touch and   Annotated further reading
  tenderness   Useful website

10   Psychological care matters   172
Introduction   The importance of the care
Chapter aims   environment
The argument for psychology in   Future challenges
  midwifery practice   References
The psychological impact of   Annotated further reading
  caring for vulnerable women

Glossary   178

Index   183

About the authors

Maureen D Raynor is a registered mental nurse, registered general nurse, midwife, midwife teacher and supervisor of midwives. She has been teaching applied behavioural sciences in the midwifery curriculum at Nottingham University for many years. Her research interests include factors influencing women's satisfaction with care, intrapartum care, perineal care, perinatal mental health and public health issues such as poverty. Nationally she is a member of the United Kingdom and Ireland Marcé Society (UKIMS), and the Perinatal Mental Health Management Group and the Maternity Services Liaison Committee (MSLC) at local level.

Carole England is a registered general nurse with a special interest in neonatal nursing and is a neonatal teacher. She is also a registered midwife and midwife teacher and is equally interested in psychology, physiology, communication and counselling.

Acknowledgements

We would like to thank all the women and families whose care experiences have been influential in shaping our understanding of psychology. Our gratitude goes to Verity for her empowering story on how independent midwifery helped to make a real difference to her experience of maternity care. Finally, we have learnt a lot about the importance of psychology from all the student midwives we have taught and midwives we have worked alongside. Last but not least our appreciation is extended to our husbands for their unconditional love, unwavering support and patience.

Acknowledgements

Introduction

Psychology and midwives

Midwives are the guardians of woman-centred care and key public health professionals at the sharp end of maternity care. Having a clear comprehension of psychology will assist midwives in understanding pregnancy, childbirth and parenthood not only as major life events but periods of adaptation and change that can result in emotional disequilibrium for women and their partners. The evidence has consistently shown that these particular developmental or transitional crises are frequently more stressful bringing about more marked changes to roles, relationships, lifestyles and family routines than any other single life event. The ease of adaptation although uniformly testing and varied, is uniquely individual. Emotional responses will be influenced by a multitude of factors including body image, interpersonal relationships, self-esteem, stress, anxiety and socio-cultural influences such as support, values and belief systems. Midwives are inimitably placed to be truly with woman, educating, informing and supporting.

This book seeks to explain the basic principles of psychology and how they relate to midwifery practice. The midwife will then be more effective in meeting women's emotional needs. Midwives are in a privileged position to meet women's psychological needs as it is widely acknowledged that midwife-led care provides women with a viable and cost-effective option (Hatem et al 2008). There is a plethora of evidence to support the theory that continuity of care and the continuous supporting role of the midwife, particularly one who the woman knows and trusts, exert a favourable outcome in the woman's satisfaction with her care. This is not only important in the woman's psychological adjustment to motherhood and her ability to mother and nurture her baby, it is central to her overall emotional wellbeing. The Care Quality Commission details a report from the former Healthcare Commission (HCC 2008), that a significant number of women are still not receiving one-to-one care during childbirth. The report acknowledges the additional pressure that is put on midwives and the maternity service by the significant rise in birth rate in the United Kingdom (UK), increasing by 16% since 2001. This added to the shortage of midwives mean many women in established labour miss out on one-to-one support from a named midwife.

Pregnancy and childbirth are an integral part of human existence. For a pregnant woman it is a culmination of swirling emotions and phenomenal change connected to the physical adaptation and hormonal chaos occurring in her body. Not only is pregnancy an exciting time for women, their partners and family, a time of heightened expectations, hopes, dreams and anticipation, it often signifies a journey into the unknown. This journey may be filled with contradictions, pleasant surprises and joy, punctuated by feelings of ambivalence, uncertainty, stress and anxiety. Not all pregnancies end in a good outcome, pregnancy can therefore be a period where doubt and trepidation prevail. Unsurprisingly, there are vast individual responses to the inherent cognitive, emotional, social, spiritual and psychological demands of pregnancy, labour and the puerperium.

Emotionally, most women will experience a period of ambivalence punctuated with negative and positive responses as they adjust to the demands and challenges of pregnancy. Their feelings may be magnified by their sense of control (Keeton et al 2008) and expectations, especially for first time mothers (Harwood et al 2007). **Self-esteem** is also important, Jomeen and Martin (2005) highlight the relationship between self-esteem and significant indicators of psychological distress such as depression and anxiety states. They concluded that a low self-esteem has a negative impact on health outcomes during pregnancy and the puerperium. Given that midwives have a very important role to play in public health, it is critical that they are well prepared for their role to identify the triggers that may culminate in emotional distress and psychological morbidity.

Key drivers for change

The importance of motherhood and fatherhood coupled with views of relationship within a family, the impact on family dynamics, parenting and parenting abilities are well documented and recognised at a policy level in England and Wales (Department of Health (DH) 2004, 2007). Guidelines and recommendations that have emerged from the National Institute for Health and Clinical Excellence (NICE 2007), the Scottish Intercollegiate Group Network (SIGN 2002) and the Centre for Maternal and Child Enquiries (CMACE) formerly known as the Confidential Enquiries into Maternal and Child Health (CEMACH) (Lewis 2007) all stress the importance of mental health and emotional wellbeing during the pregnancy continuum.

Purpose of the book

The main purpose of the book is to provide an overview of some of the key psychological issues affecting childbearing women. The aim is to challenge the midwife to reflect on learning and practice in order to develop effective strategies that will assist in meeting women's emotional needs. To help realise just that, reflective and problem-solving activities are a key feature of the book. Case vignettes extrapolated from real life experiences provide practical working examples and summary of key points have been integrated. Each chapter will be supported by references, annotated further reading, and useful websites where appropriate. A glossary of terms is incorporated at the end of the book to define more complex concepts.

Readers are invited to complete the reflective activity detailed below and think about how the theoretical perspectives or approaches to psychology apply to midwifery practice. Social psychology, for example, relates to individual behaviour in groups, interactions and relationships. It is essential for midwives to understand how such knowledge relates to their encounter with women and their role as active members of the multidisciplinary/ interprofessional teams.

Reflective activity

1. What is psychology?

2. How can psychology help us make sense of our world?

3. How can psychology help us to relate to others?

4. How can psychology help us understand behaviour or individual responses to a given situation or life crisis?

Book outline

Respect for the heterogeneity of women and knowledge of the individual variation and emotional journey each woman makes in response to pregnancy, labour and the puerperium is crucial. Chapter 1 provides explanations and definitions of the main theoretical approaches to psychology and explores their relevance to midwifery practice. By making links to the choice agenda (DH 2004, 2007, 2008) and discussing how midwives can contribute to women's psychological wellbeing, Chapter 2 examines the importance of the midwife–mother relationship and poses a number of reflective questions for practice. This is aimed at getting the reader to think critically of the psychological benefits of fostering a positive working relationship with women. Emphasis is placed on the emotional rewards in providing women with care that is both supportive and respectful. Chapter 3 gives an overview of the role psychology plays in the transition to parenthood. It identifies some of the necessary emotional responses or adjustment reactions to change during the childbearing continuum, acting as the precursor to Chapter 4, which is concerned with perinatal mental illness. Psychiatric disorders remain a leading cause of maternal morbidity and mortality in the UK (Lewis 2007). It is vital that midwives are suitably armed with the knowledge, understanding and skills to identify women at risk of serious mental illness, and make timely referrals.

Communication in midwifery practice is crucial for effective care and maternal satisfaction with care. Poor communication practice is perhaps the single most common reason for complaints within the National Health Services (NHS) and women's dissatisfaction with their care (HCC 2008, Redshaw et al 2007). Emotional reassurance through unbiased information, effective communication, empathetic listening and support are the key to effective helping. Chapter 5 highlights the concepts and principles of effective communication. The environment in which birth takes place and mothers and babies are cared for should be nurturing and empowering. Chapter 6 explores the complexities of the care environment, key cultural influences and considers the concept of 'emotion work' as popularised by Hunter and Deery (2009).

Stress and anxiety have implications for mother and fetus; these issues are examined in Chapter 7. Cross-culturally, the need for love, safety, proximity, protection and nurturance are universal experiences (Affolter 2004), emotional needs that are likely to be met when psychosocial support is present. Psychosocial support is a major determinant of health and wellbeing. Chapter 8 explores the emotional dimensions of support, its importance in forming safe and secure relationships and how it benefits women psychologically by helping to ameliorate stress, anxiety and social adversity. Emphasis is placed on how support may result in relationship discord in families and impact on the cognitive and behavioural development of children. Chapter 9 focuses on attachment theories, outlining how the quality of social experiences determines the programming of the brain and the consequences for fetal and infant development. Chapter 10 concludes the book by spelling out why psychology matters in contemporary midwifery practice.

Notes

1. Throughout the book for ease of reference and where applicable, the male is implied whenever the female gender is employed.
2. From 31 March 2009 the Healthcare Commission in England became the Care Quality Commission.
3. From July 2009 CEMACH (Confidential Enquiries into Maternal and Child Health) became CMACE (Centre for Maternal and Child Enquiries).

References

Affolter, F.W. (2004) Socio-emotionally intelligent development politics: towards a framework for socio-emotionally intelligent politics – a concept/advocacy paper. *International Journal of Psychosocial Rehabilitation*, 8: 119–40.

Department of Health (2004) *National Service Framework for Children, Young People and Maternity Services*. London: DH.

Department of Health (2007) *Maternity Matters: Access and continuity of care in a safe service*. London: DH.

Department of Health (2008) *High Quality Care for All: NHS next stage review final report* (Chair Lord Darzi). www.dh.gov.uk (accessed 28 August 2008).

Harwood, K., McLean, N. and Durkin, K. (2007) First time mothers' expectations of parenthood: what happens when optimistic expectations are not matched by later experiences? *Developmental Psychology*, 43(1): 1–12.

Hatem, M., Sandall, J., Devane, D., Soltani, H. and Gates, S. (2008) Midwife-led versus other models of care for childbearing women. *Cochrane Database of Systematic Reviews*. Art No: CD004667. DOI: 10.10021/14651858.

Healthcare Commission (2008) *Towards Better Births: a review of maternity services in England*. http://www.cqc.org.uk (accessed 12 April 2009).

Hunter, B. and Deery, R. (eds) (2009) *Emotions in Midwifery and Reproduction*. Basingstoke: Macmillan.

Jomeen, J. and Martin, C.R. (2005) Self-esteem and mental health during early pregnancy. *Clinical Effectiveness in Nursing*, 9(1–2): 92–5.

Keeton, C.P., Perry-Jenkins, M. and Sayer, A.G. (2008) Sense of control predicts depressive and anxious symptoms across the transition to parenthood. *Journal of Family Psychology*, 22(2): 212–21.

Lewis, G. (ed.) (2007) *The Confidential Enquiry into Maternal and Child Health (CEMACH). Saving mothers' lives: reviewing maternal deaths to make motherhood safer 2003–2005. The seventh report on Confidential Enquiries into Maternal Deaths in the United Kingdom*. London: CMACE.

National Institute for Health and Clinical Excellence (2007) *Antenatal and Postnatal Mental Health: clinical management service guidance, CG45*. London: NICE.

Redshaw, M., Rowe, R., Hockley, C. and Brocklehurst, P. (2007) *Recorded Delivery: a national survey of women's experience of maternity care 2006*. Oxford: National Perinatal Epidemiology Unit.

Scottish Intercollegiate Guidelines Network (2002) *Postnatal Depression and Puerperal Psychosis*. SIGN Publication No.60. www.sign.ac.uk. (accessed 1 February 2009).

Annotated further reading

Bergström, M., Kieler, H. and Waldenström, U. (2009) Effects of natural childbirth preparation versus standard antenatal education on epidural rates, experience of childbirth and parental stress in mothers and fathers: a randomised controlled multicentre trial. *British Journal of Obstetrics and Gynaecology*; DOI:10.1111/j-1471-0528.2009.02144.x. (accessed 30 May 2009).

This Swedish study provides some food for thought on the psychosocial preparation of women to achieve natural childbirth.

1 Theoretical approaches to psychology and their application to midwifery practice

Chapter contents

Introduction

Chapter aims

The major approaches to psychology

Psychologies that have evolved from the five
major approaches

Alternative approaches to psychology

Conclusion

Summary of key points

References

Annotated further reading

Useful website

Introduction

Psychology as a subject discipline is wide-ranging and complex but currently no single theory can effectively explain all its aspects. This chapter is designed to apply relevant approaches of psychology to midwifery practice. It will initially present the five major approaches in order of their historical appearance. These are behaviourism, psychoanalysis, cognitive psychology, humanistic psychology and biopsychology. From these, social and developmental psychology have evolved. Developmental psychology emphasises attachment formation and how people cope at different stages of their lifespan; social psychology focuses on the nature and cause of how people behave when in the company of others in social situations. Abnormal psychology will refer to perinatal mental illness and will be briefly discussed. More recent approaches in psychology include health psychology, social constructionism and feminism.

Chapter aims

- To present the five major approaches of psychology which are the behaviourist approach, the psychoanalytic approach, the cognitive approach, the humanistic approach and the biopsychological approach

- To explore social, developmental and abnormal approaches and how they utilise aspects of the five main approaches, to structure and define them

- To discuss the biopsychosocial model of health psychology and the health/illness continuum

- To reflect upon the social constructionist approach and its links to other psychological approaches especially feminist psychology

- To explore how each approach has application to midwifery practice
- To assert that midwifery practice can be enhanced by psychology

The major approaches to psychology

The behaviourist approach

Behavourists stress the use of defining concepts in terms of observable, measurable events. They emphasise the role of environment factors in influencing behaviour to the near exclusion of innate or inherited factors. This amounts essentially to a focus on learning.

Classical conditioning is referred to as stimulus-response psychology because it demonstrates observable behaviour (response) in terms of environmental events (stimuli). So when the midwife observes heavy lochia in a postnatal woman (stimulus), she will respond by rubbing up a contraction (conditioned response). The midwife has learned this by pairing these two events over many occasions so that her behaviour becomes predictable and automatic.

By comparison operant conditioning focuses upon how behaviour is shaped and maintained by its *consequences*. These operations are called positive reinforcement, negative reinforcement and punishment. Both positive and negative reinforcement strengthen behaviour (make it more probable), punishment weakens behaviour. If the midwife compliments a mother for the way she changed her baby's nappy, the mother's behaviour will be strengthened by this positive reinforcement. If the midwife finds the baby unattended on the mother's bed, she may choose to reprimand the mother. This approach is punishment. The mother will learn the lesson, but may feel humiliated, even angry. Alternatively, the midwife could quietly talk to her about the dangers of her baby falling to the floor (removal of an unwelcome consequence). This latter situation is an example of negative reinforcement and will strengthen the mother's behaviour (I have been lucky this time and will never do that again). Both classical and operant conditioning are forms of associative learning whereby connections are formed between stimuli and responses that did not exist before learning took place and will be influenced by context and communication style. Midwives are educators and in using appropriate psychology they can enhance their effectiveness in what can be a challenging circumstance. It is never easy to tell a person they have made an error.

The psychoanalytic approach

Founded by Sigmund Freud this approach has two major components:

- A complete account of human personality. He specified the basic structures of personality, the forces which motivate behaviour and the developmental sequence through which adult personality is acquired. Adult behaviour is determined by unconscious forces, to which a person has no conscious access.
- Psychoanalysis allows the patient access to their unconscious conflicts, motives and fears which have their origins in childhood experiences.

Freud's theory of consciousness

Freud believes that consciousness is divided into two main parts:

1. The conscious mind which contains thoughts and feelings of which there is immediately awareness at any given moment.

2. The subconscious mind which is below the level of conscious awareness and is divided into two levels:
   - the preconscious mind contains all thoughts, memories and emotions of which a person is not presently aware but can be brought into the conscious mind by deliberate choice
   - the unconscious mind contains ideas, experiences and feelings which are blocked from conscious awareness by a process of repression. Some content can leak out through random thoughts, images or dreams but Freud believes it is the unconscious mind that can be a source of disruption to mental health.

According to Freud, the mind consists of three parts:

1. The Ego, which is the practical part of the person and acts as the interface between the mind and reality.
2. The Superego is the social sense of duty, responsibility and conscience. These are found mainly in the preconscious mind (see Figure 1.1).
3. The Id is the source of all basic drives and buried desires. It demands instant gratification, is totally unconscious, but it is possible to deduce its existence when impulses break through into consciousness in slips of the tongue, symbolic dreams and psychological anxiety.

Both the Superego and Id are equally demanding in attempting to influence the Ego. Freud believes that anxiety arises when the Ego is faced with stimuli with which it cannot cope, as a result of either external danger or the demands of the Id or Superego. Defence mechanisms exist to protect the Ego from anxiety, but do so in ways that distort reality. They operate by allowing gratification in some indirect way. The Ego will often use a combination of them rather than a single mechanism (see Case vignette 1.1 and Box 1.1).

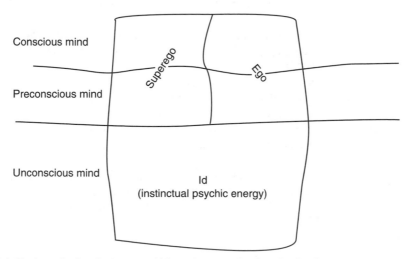

Figure 1.1 To show the Ego, Superego and Id in relation to the three levels of consciousness (adapted from Glassman and Hadad 2009; Gross 2005).

Case vignette 1.1

Amanda has an essay to write but is having difficulty in getting started. Amanda knows she has two days off duty (the Ego) and accepts that she must pass the essay to complete her module (the Superego). She wants to scream and cry (Id) but instead of making a start on her essay, she sublimates her frustrations into extensively cleaning her flat.

Box 1.1 Defence mechanisms and behaviour (adapted from Glassman and Hadad 2009; Gross 2005)

Name	Definition	Midwifery example
Denial	Refusing to acknowledge anxiety-provoking thoughts or impulses	Josie refused to accept that she was pregnant until she saw her baby on ultrasound scan
Displacement	Redirecting drive energy from one object to a substitute object	Maria is annoyed that her manager has found fault with her work and is verbally abusive about the late arrival of her new student midwife
Identification	Incorporating aspects of another person, making them part of oneself	Jane wants to become like her own mother, now that she is a mother herself
Projection	Attributing one's unacceptable thoughts and impulses onto others	'I do not like you, because you do not like me'
Rationalization	Explaining one's behaviour by offering an acceptable reason instead of the true reason	'I am sorry I am later than expected, there has been an emergency' (true reason the midwife was chatting to a colleague)
Reaction Formation	Reacting in a way that is opposite to one's actual feelings and impulses	Lauren resents and dislikes her midwife manager but acts in a friendly warm way towards her
Regression	Reverting to behaviours of gratification at an earlier stage of development	The stress of caring for her crying baby prompts Lisa to start smoking again
Repression	Blocking thoughts, memories or impulses from the conscious mind	During her booking interview, Judie fails to remember that she was abused as a child
Sublimation	Redirecting drive energy into a socially acceptable activity	Marilyn over-exerts herself at work to forget the argument she had on leaving home that morning

The Id wins out in this situation because Amanda knows that having a clean flat will make her feel good (instant gratification) whereas by comparison, the essay is perceived as a source of concern and uncertainty. By using a defence mechanism she has, according to Freud, protected her Ego from undue anxiety.

Many of the assumptions of the psychoanalytic approach have been questioned by modern psychology, including the clinical evidence upon which the whole structure is based (Webster 1995). However, according to Gross (2005) many things in life are accepted even though they cannot be tested, and psychoanalytic theories have inspired more empirical research in the social and behavioural sciences, than any other group of theories. Freud remains a dominating figure. Many mental health practitioners, including psychotherapists, counsellors and social workers incorporate elements of Freudian thought and technique into their approaches.

Application of psychoanalytic theory is widespread in midwifery practice and ranges from theories of child development, especially the development of attachment with significant others (Chapter 9), to how previous experiences may affect a mother in different ways. If a mother has had a bad experience in a previous pregnancy, she may be affected by thoughts and memories that she has tried to forget. A woman who is becoming a mother for the first time may have memories of being mothered herself and may be affected in how she perceives her present feelings, thoughts and experiences. Where anxiety exists and defence mechanisms are used, these processes may create elements of irrational behaviour, which may manifest in certain unwarranted or unpredictable communication styles (Chapters 5 and 7). The midwife could stereotype these behaviours as the emotional turmoil of pregnancy and disregard them, or she may offer the mother an opportunity to talk about her thoughts and feelings in an attempt to further understand and help her. (Psychoanalytic psychologists include Bowlby 1969, Winnicott 1990, Raphael-Leff 2005.)

Reflective activity 1.1

Think about the words that exist in everyday language that have come from psychoanalytic theory. They may include the unconscious mind, Ego, denial.

Next time you make a Freudian slip, think how it might represent a minor eruption of your unconscious processing. What does it say about you?

Which defence mechanisms do you knowingly use?

The cognitive approach

The human brain is not like other organs of the body because looking at its structure does not reveal anything about how it functions. Thus cognitive psychologists are forced to seek analogies and metaphors when trying to describe a construct within the brain. The most dominant and compelling construct compares the human mind to the computer and asserts that human behaviour is determined by interpretation of events based on incoming information and knowledge of past events, which are mentally represented. The process of analysis and the way in which knowledge is represented is now accepted and higher-order mental activities, which cannot be directly seen but are inferred, include attention, memory, perception, thinking, problem solving, reasoning, concept attainment and language.

Many situations and issues in the midwifery context are not the events themselves but the way each person perceives them (West and Bramwell 2006). Communication failures are often related to attention deficits, problems with comprehension and language difficulties. Where stress and anxiety exist, the cognitive appraisal of threat and use of coping strategies may affect thinking, decision-making and memory. The midwife must be aware of these processes and how they could be affecting the woman she is caring for. The midwife herself needs to be aware that she too can be similarly affected and disruptions to cognition will influence non-verbal communication and self-awareness.

The humanistic approach

Described by Maslow (1970) as the third force in psychology, humanistic psychology defines the person as unique, free, rational, self-determining and not controlled by stimulus–response reactions or incapacitated by unconscious motives. The person has an ability to accept and express one's true nature, to take responsibility for one's own actions and to make authentic choices. People are interpreters of themselves and their world. Behaviour is understood in terms of the person's subjective experience from their perspective, therefore the approach is one of phenomenology which means that the person is the expert on themselves. Present experience is seen as important as past experience.

Maslow's theory is based on personality development and motivation and sees self-actualisation as the peak of a *hierarchy of needs* (see Figure 1.2). Maslow's model lacks empirical evidence to lay claim to whether people can actually self-actualise, but the model is a useful conceptual framework that encapsulates many of the needs and values that are intrinsic to the psychological context of care. Maslow (1970) asserts that to progress up the hierarchy, those at the base should be initially satisfied.

Reflective activity 1.2 The Hierarchy of Needs model and midwifery practice

The reader may wish to work from the base of the hierarchy upwards and consider whether the Hierarchy of Needs model (Figure 1.2) is applicable to midwifery practice by examining the model from:

1. The woman's perspective. How may her experiences and perceptions of need differ in pregnancy, labour and the postnatal period?
2. The midwife's perspective when working in a busy antenatal/postnatal clinic, labour ward or postnatal ward. Which needs are fulfilled, which ones may get neglected?
3. The student midwife's perspective and where her needs may resonate, when working with the above people.
4. The woman's family who have their own individual and diverse set of needs.

Some needs are fundamental for survival, others are desirable and still others are exceptional if achieved. The birthing of one's baby may represent a once-in-a-lifetime experience of symmetry and beauty for some parents. For another woman, attaching her baby to the breast and seeing him suckle may meet an esteem need, long sought after. Falling short on a physiological need like rest and recuperation may totally wipe out the hierarchy for another person and create a bad day for those in her vicinity. The midwife, working all day without a comfort break, according to the humanistic approach, is engaging in reckless behaviour. She knows what is best for her and ultimately her behaviour becomes self-defeating.

The main focus of humanistic psychology is the person's sense of self. Rogers (1951) developed the concept of the *therapeutic relationship* which he incorporated into a new approach in therapy he called *client-centred therapy*. He later changed the name to *person-centred therapy* as he wanted to remove the implication of the professional power of the therapist. Both Maslow and Rogers based their principles in holism, the psychology of the whole person not disparate parts of behaviour, and this view is consistent with the holistic model of midwifery that sees the woman in terms of an integration of her mind, body and soul. Thus the core

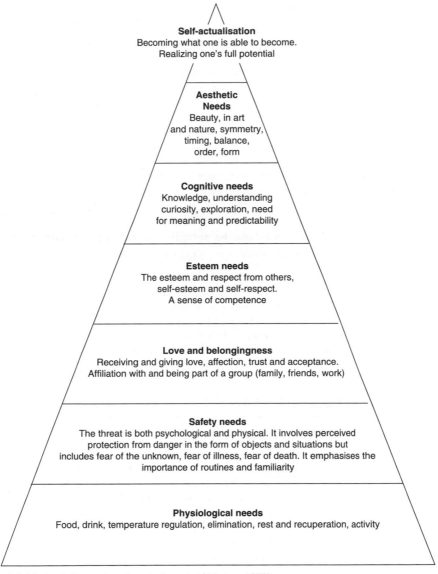

Figure 1.2 Maslow's hierarchy of needs (based on Maslow 1970).

Source: adapted from Maslow, A. (1970) *Motivation and personality.* New York. Harper and Rowe. PP, 35–38, 39–43, 182–183, 250, 275–276

conditions of the Rogerian approach are utilised by midwives to support women and their families, in many different aspects of childbearing. It is acknowledged that the midwife is not a counsellor per se but uses *counselling skills* in her role (see Chapter 5). She can offer careful and accurate listening skills, while showing empathy, acceptance (unconditional positive regard) and honesty (congruence). By adopting these *attitudes of thought and ways of being*, midwives are better prepared to offer care that is woman-centred (Rogers 1985).

The biopsychological approach

This approach seeks to understand the *physiological and genetic basis* of behaviour. Thoughts and actions find their basis in the structure of the central nervous system, especially the brain (see Box 1.2). This approach had been widely influenced by the mapping and sequencing of the human genome completed ahead of schedule in 2003. Recent developments in scanning technology such as functional magnetic resonance imaging (fMRI) have also created great advances in understanding how different parts of the brain work together (see Chapter 7). It has been shown that the limbic system, known as the emotional brain, is highly sensitive during pregnancy, labour and the puerperium. Activation of the amygdala for interpretation of facial expression and tone of voice, the hippocampus (recall of memories) and the olfactory nerves (sense of smell) can stimulate the hypothalamus, pituitary gland and autonomic nervous system to respond in accordance with incoming stimuli (Pinel 2006). This may range from a feeling of uneasiness to a major stress reaction.

Box 1.2 To show the different neuro-scientific disciplines that contribute to the biosychological approach (adapted from Pinel 2006)

- Neuro-anatomy – the structure of the nervous system
- Neuro-chemistry – the chemical basis of neural activity
- Neuro-endocrinology – interactions between the nervous system and the endocrine system
- Neuro-pathology – the study of nervous disorders
- Neuro-pharmacology – the effects of medicines and drugs on neural activity
- Neuro-physiology – functions and activities of the nervous system

Psychologies that have evolved from the five major approaches

The developmental psychology approach

This area of psychology studies the physical, intellectual, social and emotional changes that occur in a person over time, particularly the first two decades, and includes stages of child development (Glassman and Hadad 2009). The central theme is the development of meaningful attachments, which are intense, enduring emotional ties to specific people, with the mother–child relationship acting as a template for later relationships. This approach is particularly pertinent to midwifery practice because the midwife is central in attempting to foster mother–baby, father–baby relationships and prevent, where necessary, interruptions or separations to the processes involved. The psychosocial transition of motherhood involves how women react to the changes that occur when one becomes a parent. From the psychoanalytic approach, Erikson (1980) describes transitions as either normative or idiosyncratic. Normative transitions occur in accordance to the norms of one's society, will affect many people and is an experience that is largely expected (having a term baby in one's 20s with no complications). By comparison, if the transition is idiosyncratic, this only applies to the individual (birthing a stillborn baby). Idiosyncratic transitions are unexpected, stressful and psychological recovery tends to be more prolonged.

The social psychology approach

According to McKinlay and McVittie (2008) social psychology is the study of how people think, feel, desire and act in social situations. It is often said that all psychology is social psychology since all behaviour takes place in a social context; even when people are alone, their behaviour continues to be influenced by others. One's own self-concept is in large measure a reflection of this process. Interpersonal perception (how one forms impressions of others) is implicit in how women and their named midwife develop a rapport and share mutually supportive communications with each other (Chapter 5). See Case vignette 1.2.

Case vignette 1.2

Lorna was worried about her baby. He was bringing back most of each feed and seemed floppy compared to her first baby. As a healthcare professional herself she did not want to trouble the midwife as she appeared busy with other demanding women. When the midwife did approach her, she treated her like a colleague. Lorna felt unable to communicate her fears.

This social situation rendered Lorna unable to express herself as the midwife had stereotyped her as a coping mother with minimal requirements. Treating Lorna as a healthcare professional rather than a mother had altered their social roles, which also impacted on Lorna's ability to ask for help. It is important for the midwife to offer psychosocial support, even to those who appear not to need it, especially given the busy, noisy social environment in hospital. A baby with poor muscle tone that is vomiting needs paediatric referral and had the midwife offered Lorna an opportunity to talk through her fears, the midwife could have initiated the necessary neonatal care earlier and provided more focused social support to Lorna.

The abnormal psychology approach

Abnormal psychology studies the underlying causes of mental illness, behaviour disorders, emotional disturbances and forms of deviancy. According to Oates and Raynor (2009), when applied to childbearing, the term perinatal psychiatric disorder or perinatal mental illness emphasises the importance of psychiatric disorders that occur in *pregnancy* as well as those following childbirth. When a woman with a pre-existing mental illness finds out she is pregnant she may stop her medication and this may lead to recurrence or relapse of her condition. Pregnancy itself may trigger mental illness. Midwives using a holistic model need to understand what psychosocial factors may affect a woman and be able to recognise, know and understand the different types of psychiatric disorders and their management. They are divided into serious mental illnesses, mild to moderate psychiatric disorders, adjustment in reactions to life events, substance misuse, personality disorders and learning disabilities. The importance of mental health issues and the effects of morbidity and mortality on family life cannot be over-emphasised.

Alternative approaches to psychology

The health psychology approach

Health psychology pulls together educational, scientific and professional contributions to the discipline of psychology to promote and maintain health and prevent illness. It is more interested in normal psychological processes in relation to health and illness than psychiatric disorders. According to Ogden (2007), illness is caused by a combination of biological, psychological and social factors, which reflect a bio-psychosocial model of health and illness (see Box 1.3). Health and illness are not qualitatively different, but exist on a continuum and people move up and down the continuum as their health status fluctuates. Their day-to-day status is reliant upon their perception of how they feel.

Box 1.3 The biopsychosocial model of health and illness (adapted from Ogden 2007)

Bio	Psycho	Social
Genetic	Stress	Social norms of behaviour
Viruses	Pain	Social values on health
Bacteria	Emotions	Social class
Injuries	Behaviours	Ethnicity
Structural defects	Beliefs	Disability
	Coping	Employment
	Expectations	Pressures to change

Concepts such as pain and stress fit into the biopsychosocial model. Although pain is basic-ally physiological, the pain experience has emotional, cognitive and cultural components. Likewise, the causes of stress may be physical as in disruption of circadian rhythms for shift workers (biological) and occupational-linked stressors especially for healthcare workers who have little control over their workload (psychosocial). The psychology of stress has evolved from biological and social perspectives and the transactional model sees stress as the fit between a person and their environment and whether they feel they can cope. Coping with threat involves primary and secondary appraisal and utilisation of approach-focused and/or avoidance-focused coping strategies. Threats to the self-concept can result in negative emotions that may adversely affect health (Klaus and Lebherz 2008).

Barlow et al (2008) report on women who were in hospital for hypertension during preg-nancy and comment on how some women felt a fraud in occupying a bed when they had no symptoms of ill health. These women searched for meaning of their situation, in an attempt to adapt to an unexpected, threatening event. This paradox prevented some women from willingly accepting care such as bed rest and medication. The authors agree that the midwife could help such women by affirming their status as worthy of hospital care. The provision of consistent, easily understood information on a regular basis is also recommended with the provision of opportunity to talk about how they feel. Social support from midwives, fellowship with other women on the ward, and family can help them feel more accepted and less confused. This study reflects how health psychology in rejecting the mind–body split, supports the *whole person* approach to health. The mind is thought to be involved in both the cause and treatment of illness and supports the view that each person is responsible for their own health and is not a passive victim. See Case vignette 1.3.

Case vignette 1.3

Vivien was 28 weeks pregnant, financially comfortable but complained that she was 'hooked on junk food' and feared for her baby's health. She was physically healthy but she said she 'knew she was doing wrong' and felt guilty.

The midwife's role in health promotion in this antenatal clinic situation is to encourage behaviour change in providing Vivien with relevant information to enable her to change her attitude to her eating choices and how to choose coping strategies that will enable her to feel better about herself and cause less harm to her and her growing fetus. The midwife at this juncture could give Vivien a lecture on what she should be eating, however it is argued that Vivien's compliance to change her behaviour will be affected by how the midwife communicates her own beliefs to her (how convincing she is) and Vivien's sense of satisfaction with the interaction. Crucial to this process is Vivien's desire to change and her cognitive ability to understand, recall and personally connect with the information provided. Given the time constraints on the midwife, the most effective way for her is to find out what Vivien eats and what she feels she should eat. The midwife can then facilitate Vivien in creating her own goals and targets, which can be followed up with each future visit. In taking responsibility for her own actions, Vivien is more likely to be compliant with her own health agenda and given there is some continuity of care, the midwife will be able to encourage and reassure her of her success (Ogden 2007).

The social constructionist (SC) approach

This approach argues that all knowledge, which includes psychological knowledge, is historically and culturally specific and the way to study the person must include their social, political and economic realms of life. The midwife who is taking a booking history from a woman who is a newly arrived migrant must consider her in terms of these features and how she has been affected by her experiences. Since the only common feature of social life is that it is continually changing, all one can do is to try to understand and account for how her world appears at this present time. MacLachlan (2004) asserts that when people from different cultures interact, understandings of reality may differ. Burr (2003) argues that there is no recognition of *essentials* such as behaviourism or cognitive psychology, because these are based on the ideas of some pre-given ability of the person, so in turn the nature/ nurture debate is also rejected. Furthermore, any theories and explanations of psychology which are time and culture bound, cannot be taken as once-and-for-all descriptions of human nature.

It is further argued that language is a precondition for thought and people are born into a world where the conceptual frameworks and categories used in one's culture already exist. When people talk to each other the world gets constructed, so language is a form of social action. The way the midwife uses language will construct meaning for the woman in her care, even if she only understands that the world she has entered is very different to her own. Therefore in SC, people construct their own and others' identities through their everyday encounters with each other in social interaction and, in so doing, their own versions of reality.

According to SC, language is constructed into a series of discourses. A discourse refers to a set of meanings, metaphors, representations, images, stories or statements that in some way produce a particular version of events. Each discourse claims to be the truth. So when an issue is said to be socially constructed, it comes from this stance. When a midwife works in a culture where discourses constantly focus on poor care, loss of job satisfaction, stress, disillusionment, poor leadership, this becomes her reality.

Social constructionism and feminist psychology

Discourses construct social phenomena in different ways. Some appear to receive the label of truth or common sense more readily than others and this is directly related to power. Discourses are intimately connected to the way that society is organised and run, so in a capitalist economy dominated by men, the law, education, religion, marriage and family all give shape and substance to each person's daily life which provides different levels of status and social position.

Discourse socially constructs motherhood as a vital aspect of femininity. Women often engage with the ideal image of motherhood, but find its reality quite different (Choi et al 2005, Weaver and Ussher 1997).

The feminist approach

McKinlay and McVittie (2008) assert that some of the most influential theories within psychology are based on studies of males only, but are meant to apply equally to both women and men. If women's behaviour differs from men's the former is often judged through gender discourses to be pathological, abnormal or deficient in some way (sexism) and this is because the behaviour of men is implicitly and explicitly taken as the standard against which women's behaviour is compared. Traditional explanations of behaviour emphasise that sex differences are biologically determined and not socially constructed. This view reinforces widely held stereotypes held by men and women, about men and women, which contributes to the oppression of women. In the same way, heterosexuality (both male and female) is taken as the norm so that homosexuality is seen as abnormal.

Case vignette 1.4

Julie and Jane decided to have a baby together. Julie became pregnant by artificial insemination by a known sperm donor. Two years later, Jane underwent the same process. In this same-sex couple, both women are mother to their own child and both children have the same biological father. As a family of four they are thriving.

Julie and Jane are not conventional parents but still require care that a non-judgemental midwife can offer. Feminist psychologists work to contextualise women's lives and explain the constraints within a social framework and women's lack of social power. According to Kaufmann (2004), a feminist approach supports the endorsement of equal opportunity, equal treatment, and the belief that women should be accorded their true value. Embracing feminism can help midwives to understand the diverse realities of women's lives and to support and respect each woman with whom they work. Woman-centred care is paramount to this philosophy.

Conclusion

This chapter has provided a brief overview of how psychology from certain approaches can contribute to midwifery care. Conceptually midwifery care is complex in its own way and there is no one psychological approach that can be, or should be, adopted. The five major approaches of psychology were developed largely over the 20th century and are influenced by the culture that existed at that time. Each approach represents a distinct framework for the study of behaviour and how they differ provides a way to understand the significance of each approach. More recent approaches take account of the effects of society, culture and economics on the person, particularly health psychology that has redefined health, illness, stress and pain. Social constructionism has challenged traditional psychology (based on logical empiricism) and argues for a person psychology that is primarily influenced by social processes that is not just a new theory, but a new way of seeing the world. Thus social constructionism represents a paradigm shift in psychology (Glassman and Hadad 2009). Feminism is now an accepted approach to psychology that explores through discourse analysis and other qualitative methods, the experience of motherhood from the point of view of the mother. If woman-centred care is at the heart of midwifery care this means that the midwife should engage with her as a person and honour her dignity, intellect, history and sense of self. Psychology as a subject discipline has much to offer midwives and if midwives feel able to relate to psychology, they will come to appreciate its inherent value.

Summary of key points

- The different approaches to psychology reflect the differences psychologists have in deciding what aspect of a person is worthy of study.

- Some approaches emphasise internal workings of the brain, mind/intellect whilst others consider the environment as *the* influencing agent.

- The contribution of social constructionism affirms the importance of social, cultural, environmental, political and economic aspects of people's lives. This applies to the woman, her family, the midwife and the organisation in which she works. Written and spoken discourses create for each person, the truths and realities of their experiences.

- The impact of feminist psychology positions the midwife as an enabler to communicate a positive cherishing attitude of her faith in the woman to take responsibility for her own body and her emerging parenthood role. Similarly midwives should demonstrate mutually supportive behaviours to each other and immediately vanquish any suggestions of gender stereotypes and bigotry.

- Certain approaches of psychology can make meaningful contributions to midwifery care.

References

Barlow, J.H., Hainsworth, J. and Thornton, S. (2008) Women's experiences of hospitalisation with hypertension during pregnancy: feeling a fraud. *Journal of Reproductive and Infant Psychology*, 26(3): 157–67.

Bowlby, J. (1969) *Attachment and Loss. Volume 1. Attachment.* Harmondsworth: Penguin.

Burr, V. (2003) *Social Constructionism*, 2nd edn. Hove: Routledge.

Choi, P., Henshaw, C., Baker, S. and Tree, J. (2005) Supermum, superwife, supereverything: performing femininity in the transition to motherhood. *Journal of Reproductive and Infant Psychology*, 23(2): 167–80.

Erikson E.H. (1980) *Identity and the Life Cycle.* New York: Norton.

Glassman, W.E. and Hadad, M. (2009) *Approaches to Psychology*, 5th edn. London: McGraw-Hill, pp 229–50.

Gross, R. (2005) *Psychology. The science of mind and behaviour*, 5th edn. London: Hodder and Arnold, pp 748–9.

Kaufmann, T. (2004) Introducing feminism. In: M. Stewart and S.C. Hunt (eds) *Pregnancy, Birth and Maternity Care: Feminist Perspectives.* London: Books for Midwives, pp 1–11.

Klaus, J. and Lebherz, C. (2008) Social psychology in action. In: M. Hewstone, W. Stroebe 2nd, J. Klaus (eds) *Introduction to Social Psychology. A European Perspective.* Malden: Blackwell Publishing, pp 315–44.

McKinlay, A. and McVittie, A. (2008) *Social Psychology and Discourse.* Chichester: Wiley-Blackwell.

MacLachlan, M. (2004) Culture, empowerment and health. In: M. Murray (ed.) *Critical Health Psychology.* London: Palgrave Macmillan, pp 110–17.

Maslow, A. (1970) *Motivation and Personality.* New York: Harper and Rowe.

Oates, M.R. and Raynor, M.D (2009) Perinatal psychiatric disorder. In: D.M. Frazer and M.A. Cooper (eds) *Myles Textbook for Midwives*, 15th edn. Edinburgh: Churchill Livingstone, pp 686–703.

Ogden, J. (2007) *Health Psychology.* London: McGraw-Hill.

Pinel, J.P.J. (2006) *Biopsychology*, 6th edn. London: Pearson Education.

Raphael-Leff, J. (2005) *Psychological Processes of Childbearing*. London: The Anna Freud Centre.
Rogers, C.R. (1985) Towards a more human science of the person. *Journal of Humanistic Psychology*, 25: 7–24.
Rogers, C.R. (1951) *Client-centred Therapy*. Boston: Houghton-Mifflin.
Weaver, J.J. and Ussher, J.M. (1997). How motherhood changes life: a discourse analytic study with mothers of young children. *Journal of Reproductive and Infant Psychology*, 15(1): 51–68.
Webster, R. (1995) *Why Freud was Wrong. Sin, Science and Psychoanalysis*. London: Harper Collins.
West, H. and Bramwell, R. (2006) Do maternal screening tests provide psychological meaningful results? Cognitive psychology in an applied setting. *Journal of Reproductive and Infant Psychology*, 24(1): 61–9.
Winnicott, D.W. (1990) *The Maturation Process and the Facilitating Environment*. London: Karnac Books.

Annotated further reading

Blyth, E., Burr, V. and Farrand, A. (2008) Welfare of the child assessments in assisted conception: A social constructionist perspective. *Journal of Reproductive and Infant Psychology*, 26(1): 31–43.

This article provides a guide to how social constructionists deconstruct discourse through a process of discourse analysis and shows how issues are constructed and presented for purpose.

Useful website

Mapping and Sequencing the Human genome.

www.ornl.gov/sci/TechResources/Human_Genome/home.html

2 The mother–midwife relationship

Chapter contents

Introduction

Chapter aims

Being with woman: establishing and building relationships

Constraining factors

Significant others

Conclusion

Summary of key points

References

Annotated further reading

Introduction

> The relationship that develops between the woman and the midwife is at the core of human caring and may provide the basis of the professional body of knowledge that encapsulates midwifery (Siddiqui 1999: 111).

Midwifery knowledge continues to be defined and shaped from the experiences gained from being with women, and from the very wisdom of the women midwives have established relationships with. As stated in the opening quote by Siddiqui (1999) the midwife–mother relationship is an important and symbiotic one. This is pivotal in the context of behavioural psychology, informing midwives that relationships are complex social interactions. In order to comprehend how midwives and women can form an alliance and establish a meaningful and positive relationship, a wide array of intricately woven psychosocial factors must be considered. Not least of which are how personable the midwife is, her ability to show positive regard for others, the language used, the manner in which she communicates and the levels of confidence and competence she conveys to the woman. The behaviour, personal traits and characteristics of both the midwife and woman are also important as they can impact on the dynamics of a relationship. The way in which the midwife interacts with the woman will be much more momentous when there is mutual respect and trust. The mother–midwife relationship needs time to flourish and develop allowing scope for reciprocity to be achieved (Kirkham 2000, 2009).

This chapter explores the importance of the mother–midwife relationship, suggesting that it is the thread that binds women and midwives together, and forms the essence of care, essential for women's pleasure and fulfilment as well as job satisfaction and feelings of contentment on the part of the midwife. It also considers challenges for student midwives' socialisation and constraints to the mother–midwife relationship as well as the wider pressures on midwives working within the National Health Service (NHS) that may conspire against them being truly 'with woman'. Readers are advised to read Chapter 5, which explores the importance of communication in midwifery practice to deepen their comprehension of the issues explored within this chapter.

Chapter aims

- To examine the midwife–mother relationship and the complexities involved in such dynamic encounters

- To explore the factors that contribute to midwives establishing positive working relationships with women and other members of the interprofessional team

- To discuss the importance of the midwife–mentor/student dyad and the value of this relationship

- To highlight the different dimensions of power alongside the factors in the institutional setting that might render the woman, student and midwife powerless

---

Being with woman: establishing and building relationships

A significant number of researchers account for the importance of the midwife–mother relationship (Lundgren and Berg 2007, Hunter 2006, Kirkham 2000, Lavender et al 1999, Halldorsdottir and Karlsdottir 1996). This relationship forms the basis for women's positive experience during their maternity care experience. Central to this is the quality of support the woman receives from the midwife.

The nature of human interactions means that at the first encounter during the antenatal period, the midwife should value the time she has to establish rapport with the pregnant woman. This initial encounter is precious, an important opportunity for the midwife to sow the seeds for a new relationship to flourish and grow. The midwife and woman will be making a mental assessment and formulating a mental image or impression of each other, be that good or bad. Of course in some circumstances the midwife might have had previous encounters with the woman. Indeed, some women will be so impressed by the care, clinical competence and ability of the midwife to make them feel safe and valued, that they will actively seek care from that midwife again during subsequent pregnancies. A 'good' midwife, Pembroke and Pembroke (2006) delineate, values woman and respects her individuality. This is fundamental in the hospital setting where genuine hospitality and a welcoming and warm greeting are necessary for women to feel relaxed and comfortable.

Due to the schedule of antenatal appointments (National Institute for Health and Clinical Excellence (NICE) 2008) the relationship between the woman and midwife is relatively dynamic, requiring the midwife to be responsive and flexible in order to meet the woman's changing healthcare needs as the pregnancy progresses. A familiar midwife known to the woman antenatally is the optimal model that midwives should aspire to as it makes it easier for both to relate to each other when the woman goes into labour. A respectful and positive relationship between the midwife and woman, based on partnership, can be extremely beneficial to both. In the case of the woman, the cultivation of a positive relationship with the midwife can prove supportive, enabling and sustaining during the course of pregnancy, labour and puerperium. It can also impact on progress during labour and her achievement of normality; it is common to feel safe when women can trust the environment and their carers (Smith et al 2009, O'Neill 2008). A sense of personal fulfilment and satisfaction with care is also more likely as the mother makes the transition to motherhood. The midwife too will gain a sense of achievement, pleasure and job satisfaction. This is well documented in the literature relating to those midwives who provide continuity of care with carer throughout pregnancy, labour and postpartum (Page 2003, Sandall et al 2001, McCourt et al 1998).

Kirkham (2009) highlights the importance of context in relationship building, indicating that unlike midwives who work in birth centres or midwife-led units, midwives on busy 'high tech' labour suites have evolved coping strategies to enable them to cope with the demands of their working environment. In order to survive in such settings, particularly where midwives can exercise very little choice and control over their workload, can be a traumatic experience for midwives (Kirkham 2007). Some will either leave or others will find ways of coping (Kirkham et al 2006, Ball et al 2002). Midwives who work in large labour suites are fraught when the department is busy, and have very little time to provide quality care to women. How can a midwife who is allocated two to three women at various stages of labour be truly with woman? In such instances Kirkham (2009: 235) declares that midwives develop a form of 'professional detachment' in order to 'process women through the system'. This has marked psychological implications that can affect the relationship between the woman and midwife and lead to a care deficit (see Case scenario 2.1).

Hunter and Deery (2009) explain that midwifery involves much emotional work. Unless the midwife is very skilled at containing her emotions and is self-aware, being conscious how the non-verbal cues she is exhibiting are communicated to women (see Chapters 5 and 7), woman and midwife will withdraw from the relationship as a means of coping. This risk is more likely to be elevated when the workload is frantic; childbearing women soon pick up on how pre-occupied and busy the midwife is, resulting in avoidance (Kirkham 2009). This results in reluctance on women's part to ask for help, thus stifling their needs and culminating in a form of passivity (Kirkham 2009) as women show due consideration for how demanding and hectic the midwife's workload is. A deficit of emotional skills often result in midwives 'doing to' and 'checking women' rather than being with and listening to women (Kirkham 2009, Kirkham et al 2002). Arguably there are times when the midwife is challenged in embracing 'with-woman' philosophy and will actively encourage women to have an epidural. The epidural then acts as the surrogate midwife; conversely women might opt for an epidural to maintain some element of control if they sense that the midwife is too busy to be emotionally available to them (see Case scenario 2.1).

Case scenario 2.1

Anna is in spontaneous labour at term; following spontaneous rupture of the membranes (SROM), she arrives at her local maternity unit accompanied by her partner Harrison, eagerly anticipating the arrival of their first baby. The couple had made unsuccessful attempts to notify the labour suite of their imminent arrival but the telephone line seemed perpetually engaged. Labour suite was extremely busy due to a high volume of labouring women and staff sickness. The labour suite coordinator was not best pleased about the couple's un-notified arrival and her unwelcoming greeting – 'why didn't you call? We have no beds' – served only to alienate the couple as they entered the mêlée of the labour suite. Such confrontational manner immediately created a barrier to communication, this coupled with the midwife's closed body language and stern demeanour did very little to put the couple at ease and sow the seeds for establishing meaningful relationships.

A birthing room was eventually found to accommodate Anna. The midwife who was allocated to her care read Anna's birth plan, noting silently that she wanted a natural physiological labour. To help realise this she wanted to use the birthing pool for the entire duration of her labour and birth. She also wanted to play the CDs obtained at her hyno-birthing classes to help with self-hypnosis. Harrison was to act as the conduit or gate keeper for any questions the midwife might want to explore with Anna. Typically of the large labour suite, the midwife had competing priorities, i.e. another woman in early labour to care for, and informed Anna that she could not use the birthing pool as she was unable to provide her with one-to-one care due to workload pressures. After completing the admission process the midwife was called to attend to the needs of the other woman she was caring for, who was being prepared for theatre to have an emergency caesarean section. Anna and Harrison were therefore left unattended for long periods. The named midwife did not return from theatre for almost 2 hours to resume the care of Anna. In the midwife's absence, other members of the midwifery team made periodic checks on Anna, mainly in the form of completing tasks such as routine monitoring and recording of vital signs and fetal heart rate auscultation. They too had lots of apologies but very little time to be emotionally available to Anna. Not surprisingly, upon the named midwife's return, she noted a change in both Anna's and Harrison's demeanour. Anna was tearful and looked quite distressed and fearful, whilst Harrison's sense of anger at their loss of control and powerlessness in the given situation was palpable. The midwife judged incorrectly that Anna was not 'coping' with the challenges and demands of labour and strongly recommended that Anna should have an epidural.

Reflective activity

1. How could the midwife who greeted this couple be more welcoming in her remarks?
2. Consider the commonly cited 4 Cs: choice, control, communication and continuity of care with a named midwife and assess:

   i. why they are valuable to women like Anna, satisfaction/dissatisfaction with their care
   ii. contribute to women's emotional wellbeing.

The case vignette illustrates some of the pressures and organisational issues that preclude midwives being with women, and can impact on the achievement of normality and safe outcomes for mothers and babies. Kirkham (2009) states that the labour suite can be an environment where women are assembled and processed with little regard for their emotional needs, depending on the 'busyness' of the midwife. These are issues addressed by the qualitative study by Smith et al (2009). This research explored the views of healthcare professionals about safety in the maternity services. The predominant group who responded to this research were midwives, and the results revealed stark implications for practice. In order to support women, midwives need support and should not be afraid to speak out and inform the coordinator of the shift, the supervisor of midwives and manager when staffing levels fall below a safe standard.

Safety

Smith et al (2009) report certain areas of practice that compromise safety. This extends to poor staffing levels, communication barriers, poor skill mix, inexperienced midwives feeling devalued, unsupported and generally demoralised. The over-medicalisation of childbirth, fewer midwives and a trend towards increased technology also affect midwives' ability to achieve normality for women. There are calls for revisions to the current framework, and organisation of maternity care in the NHS is needed to enhance clinical safety (Bick 2008, O'Neill 2008). Low morale creates a vicious cycle of staff sickness, 'burn out' and substandard care resulting in further demoralisation (Smith et al 2009). Midwife-led care provides a real alternative to enhance safety (Bick 2008, Hatem et al 2008). There is also strong evidence that women who are most vulnerable to psychological morbidity or have co-existing morbidities may benefit most from this model of care (Sandall et al 2001).

Trust and reciprocity

Relationships form the core of women's experience during pregnancy, labour and childbirth. Factors that can affect relationships are many and varied, including trust, environment, language, communication (verbal and non-verbal), coercion, reciprocity, cultural sensitivity and awareness as well as competence and a feeling of safety. Trust, is perhaps the key ingredient to any relationship; without trust there is no relationship as it acts as the platform from which to provide care (Powell-Kennedy et al 2004, Thornstensen 2000). Trust is the foundation of positive interpersonal or social interactions and a pivotal part of professionalism. A relationship devoid of trust affects everything. It affects the woman's willingness to engage with care, to ask questions and to be involved in decision-making. Midwives who fail to live up to women's expectations of how professional they are may be perceived as untrustworthy. Reciprocity is also vital; a relationship based on mutual regard, where there is give-and-take is more likely to achieve partnership, shared ideas and decision-making as well as trust. The need to feel safe, secure and nurtured is also highly regarded. Altman and Taylor (1973) suggest that relationship with others and the need to connect with another human being is a powerful motivational force. This has some resonance with the maxim 'no man is an island'. Women who leave the safety and security of loved ones and their own homes to be hospitalised whether during pregnancy, labour or postpartum, need to feel cherished, respected and valued. Women's experiences of pregnancy and childbirth will be coloured by their relationship with midwives; this is why case holding is such an important model of care (McCourt and Stevens 2009).

Spiritual dimension of care

Pembroke and Pembroke (2006) highlight the spiritual dimension of caring coupled with the attitudinal or behavioural traits women value in midwives and identify three dimensions of spiritual caring:

1. *Presence*: having presence means the midwife is fully engaged with the woman.
2. *Responsibility*: signifies the capacity to respond empathetically to the needs of the woman. These needs include the desire to be listened to, to be respected, supported and understood. It also involves reciprocity and the diffusion of power that supports the woman's autonomy by being conscious of language and communication. This includes behaviour and information framing. It is important for the midwife to adopt a *neutral position*. In other words she does not allow personal biases and prejudices to influence her behaviour, the woman or care decisions.
3. *Availability*: captures the essence or willingness of the midwife to give of herself, to be unselfish, to be truly 'with woman'. Pembroke and Pembroke (2006) outline two components of *availability* as being:
   a. the ability to be responsive to women's needs
   b. the ability to be calm and reassuring.

Being available, these authors conclude, is to meet the spiritual needs of women. Thus in order to achieve partnership or have a 'relational presence' with women, the midwife not only needs to be a professional friend, she also needs to be an 'anchored companion', confident in her abilities, trusting women's decisions and believing in their power and free will as independent thinkers. Pembroke and Pembroke (2006) stress that spiritual dimension of care involves the search for 'edifying values' and entails the assurance of forgoing the 'ego identity' state. Egotistical carers, they suggest, are prisoners in their own bodies; selfish and emotionally stunted individuals who are not emotionally available to help others. Midwives who are able to release their inner self or let their common humanity come to the fore are emotionally available. Often this requires the midwife to 'do less and give more' (Leap 2000). The focus should be on being rather than doing (Walsh 2006). This means being attentive, reading the woman's body language or 'communication sites'. Observing the woman's posture, breathing, eyes and general facial expressions perhaps means more than the spoken language (Pembroke and Pembroke 2006).

Mothering the mother

The centrality of the mother–midwife dyad is the key to being with woman (Hunter 2006). Pembroke and Pembroke (2006) identify that when the midwife provides the woman with her calming and nurturing presence, and her emotional availability amidst the stresses and strains of a busy labour suite (see Case scenario 2.1), she is providing the core conditions of a mother figure. This is echoed by Freeman (2006) and Walsh (2006). Women who are treated hospitably by an initial greeting by the midwife, who experience 'emotional ambience' such as being comforted, held, stroked, rocked as in a lullaby and receive one-to-one support during labour, equate such characteristics with their mother (Walsh 2006). Freeman (2006) disputes claims that continuity of carer is fundamental to midwives achieving partnership with women or being a predictor of women's satisfaction with their care. The quality of the interaction, personal attributes and interpersonal skills of the midwife, seem to far outweigh her mere physical presence. Continuity of carer is ineffective if the midwife is not emotionally available to sculpt a meaningful and respectful relationship with the woman.

Constraining factors

The structures and constraints of care within the NHS can rob midwives of the chance to use their professional judgement to work with women, share power and take responsibility for their actions as autonomous accountable practitioners. Students will often mirror the behaviour and attitudes of their mentors. Kirkham (2009) states that behaviour, feelings and emotions are modulated according to social norms as well as the importance or value attached to social relationships. The student midwife for example strives to be liked and to be accepted by her midwife mentors. This is because students need to learn in environments that are conducive to learning, and which are supportive and empowering. Hunter (2008) suggests student midwives need scope within the curriculum to explore both the science and art of midwifery. Highlighting that as a consequence of different ways of knowing during childbirth, midwifery needs 'multiple doers' as well as 'multiple knowers'.

Power and powerlessness

Knowledge is power, yet understanding power and powerlessness is complex as these are multi-dimensional and difficult concepts to define. Drawing on the field of psychotherapy, Hildebrand and Markovic (2007) present a non-pathological view of power and the inherent associated psychosocial, economic, political and cultural dimensions of power. They define power as a means of having agency or an ability to influence, respond, bring about or effect change. Their definition of powerlessness on the other hand relates to a position of helplessness, where an individual lacks agency, is devoid of ability or power to influence, respond or effect change. In other words the person becomes ineffective and lacks clout to make a difference and whose opinions are rendered invalid by those in power or with power. Hildebrand and Markovic (2007) like Foucault (2001) recognise the negative and positive forces of power (Figure 2.1). Negative power provides a narrow perspective as it can be oppressive, repressive inhibitive and prohibitive at the same time. Conversely positive power has the ability to be a liberating, constructive and self-affirming force.

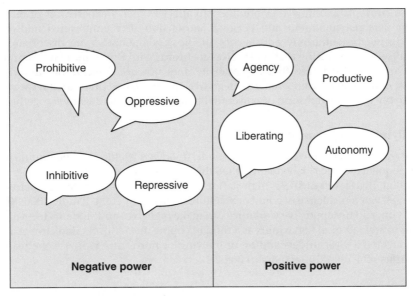

Figure 2.1 Negative and positive aspects of power

Power motivates an individual behavioural system to take risks to achieve their outcomes. Some women such as those who embrace **free birthing** choose to assert the validity of their own ways of knowing and being, firmly believing in the power of their own bodies to nurture, protect and birth their babies unassisted. These women choose to be free of the growing **hegemony** or mainstream epistemological approach of what they construe to be dominance by the all powerful medical establishment who may usurp their power and deny their choice and control during pregnancy/childbirth. Hence it can be seen that legitimate power or organisation power, provides the healthcare professional with the right or authority to preside over others and influence their decision-making. Equally, illegitimate power that exceeds authority or is motivated by self-interest can result in conflict and lead to resistance from women and the workforce, even when those individuals are considered powerless.

Psychologically, powerlessness creates a form of inertia. Where power motivates an individual's behavioural approach to take action, powerlessness often results in inaction by inhibiting or restricting the individual to take action and to be effective. This is a form of oppression. Theoretical approaches to power and oppression such as Freire's (1993: 90) work on 'pedagogy of the oppressed' underlines the dominant hegemony of particular groups who are able to oppress others: 'Only as the oppressed discover themselves to be hosts of the oppressor can they contribute to the midwifery of their liberating pedagogy. Liberation is thus a childbirth and a painful one.'

Commenting on the pressures on midwives in the NHS, an editorial by Kirkham (2003) implies that midwives are 'the shock absorbers' of an overstretched, under-resourced, medicalised, inadequate and inequitable service. A feature of powerlessness she concludes is linked to oppression. Furthermore, powerlessness and depression are intertwined and oppression and depression deskill and devalue midwives, sapping their motivation and ability to effect change.

Foucault (2001) saw all human relationships as being to some degree a power relation. He provides a fluid approach to how power is conceptualised. An empowered midwife understands power dynamics, recognises the potential for powerlessness. She acknowledges the interplay of these concepts and how they are likely to affect women's experiences of maternity care and their personal fulfilment and personal satisfaction. The empowered midwife also aims to maximise the autonomy and agency of those women who are disenfranchised and marginalised by advocating that their voices are heard. With this in mind it is central to the essence of woman-centred care that the midwife does not use coercive or authoritative power to leech control away from women. Integrative power is based on mutual respect and trust and is arguably the strongest form of power that binds midwives and women together.

Bullying or horizontal violence

The ways in which power is acquired, understood and wielded will determine its psychological consequences. There is evidence that the co-existence of low morale, role ambiguity, role conflict, high levels of stress, high staff sickness and poor job satisfaction permeate when there is an elevated incidence of a bullying culture (Curtis et al 2006, Randle 2006, Kirkham 1999). A bullying and unsupportive workforce can make midwives and students feel vulnerable and can lead to stereotypical behaviours as a form of coping mechanism (Stapleton et al 2002a, 2002b). To develop a clear understanding of bullying or horizontal violence the reader is invited to complete the reflective activity in Box 2.1.

Box 2.1 Reflective activity

- Provide your own working definition for the term bullying/horizontal violence.
- What are the signs of bullying behaviour?
- How can bullying in the workplace affect: (a) the individual? (b) the team?
- Have you ever been the subject of bullying or observed others being bullied? Reflect on how this made you feel.
- Identify the actions you would take to challenge bullying behaviour.

Significant others

Student midwives' emotional journey

Many students enter midwifery with great commitment, intrinsic motivation, drive and enthusiasm. However, it is not unusual for many to become less enthused and quickly disillusioned when the harsh reality of care within the NHS fails to live up to their expectations. The way in which current midwifery education is delivered must take into consideration the culture, structure and organisation of care in the NHS as well as the opportunities, constraints and threats to the midwife's role. The work of Hunter and Deery (2009) illustrates the emotion work involved in midwifery practice that should be built into pre-registration midwifery programmes. The recently revised standards on pre-registration midwifery issued by the Nursing and Midwifery Council (NMC 2009) state the kind and content that must be included in the curriculum for student midwives, with emphasis placed on woman-centred care. Moreover the expectation is for opportunities to be available to ensure students develop sound knowledge, comprehension and practice based competencies of the spiritual, psychosocial and emotional dimensions of care. Rule 6 of the *Midwives Rules and Standards* (NMC 2004) guiding principle is that midwifery education should provide student midwives with a wide range of experience, including the provision of midwifery care in the domiciliary setting. Home births or births in a midwife-led unit, for example, provide good working examples of the midwife being truly with woman (see Chapter 6 for Verity's story). This will ensure that on successful completion of a programme of education, the registered midwife is able to assume responsibility and account-ability for her practice in any setting. It is essential that all efforts are made to give student midwives experience of intrapartum care in home settings. Teaching should also account for how these factors may contribute to positive and negative consequences for 'normal physiology'. This should extend to the importance of fostering and cultivating effective interpersonal skills, including those of self-awareness and communication. Siddiqui (1999) charges midwife educators with the task of ensuring student midwives are *au fait* with the central tenets of caring, building and maintaining a therapeutic relationship with women. This she states should be at the core of any midwifery curriculum.

Seeing and knowing

The socialisation of student midwives forms a pivotal part in their journey to becoming autonomous, accountable midwives, acting as the axis or driver to the values and beliefs that become deeply rooted about childbearing women (Yearsley 1999). The ways in which students view their world, observe, see, gain knowledge and experience, and question practice will influence their interpretation and the sense they make of professional practice (Thornstensson et al 2008). This is integral to decision-making, clinical judgement and the way they respond and communicate in a given situation. If the traditional meaning of a midwife is 'being with woman' then the way in which students are socialised will have a profound bearing on how they view others and themselves, not only as women, but as future midwives. The qualities they think a midwife should have and how they observe midwives being with women instead of *doing to* or *for women* (Page 2003) will also have an impact.

A number of studies have highlighted the tremendous emotional investment students make to practice settings and the whole process of learning in order to feel part of the team and to navigate relationships with midwives (Jones and Wylie 2008, Thornstensson et al 2008). These studies identify role modelling as being the nexus to how students learn to be supportive, gain confidence and competence in their skills and abilities, and how they perceive their role in the interprofessional team. Earlier studies such as Begley (2001a, 2001b) and Davies and Atkinson (1991) identified that students want to feel valued and part of the team. Many develop coping strategies to enable them to fit in and feel accepted. Yearsley (1999) reported students adopting subservient roles and behaviours such as making tea or 'doing the obs' to facilitate a form of acceptance. A learning environment that fails to provide evidence based care and immerse students in an environment of work or 'just doing the obs' creates confusion and unhappiness for students (Davies and Atkinson 1991). This increases their fear and anxiety and sense of vulnerability. Students' perception of being thrown in at the deep end to sink or swim, Begley (2001b) warns, might be construed as 'character building' to some midwives, but the education of students should take precedence as it is a worthwhile investment to ensure future midwives who have developed the toolkit to establish autonomous practice and care for women sensitively.

Student midwives' lived realities or experience of pregnancy, labour and childbirth will shape their personal philosophies. The richness and diversity of such experiences, however, are not always beneficial to women. Thompson (2005) argues that this may be a source of tension and conflict not only between midwives but with the very women they serve. This is notable when pregnancy and childbirth are viewed from different standpoints or, as outlined in Chapter 6, there are competing ideologies and approaches at play, for example social model of care versus technocratic or medical model.

Midwife–doctor relationship

Cameron and Taylor (2007) assert that the unpredictable nature of pregnancy and childbirth require midwives to contract alliances with other allied health professionals. Midwives and doctors are perhaps the group that work most frequently together. Midwives work cooperatively and collaboratively with an array of different disciplines both in the community and hospital settings including general practitioners, specialist community nurses/health visitors, obstetricians, anaesthetists, neonatologists/paediatricians, physicians, surgeons, physiotherapists, psychiatrists, psychologists and specialist nurses. Historically the midwife–doctor relationship has been the source of much tension and conflict in maternity care, and is perhaps the most significant as it has implications for women's choice and outcomes (Cameron and Ellwood 2006). The midwife–doctor relationship is pivotal in maternity care as this is a relationship that can be hampered by power dynamics and subverted by the struggle for control over pregnancy and childbirth. In a provocative and thought-provoking article, Dornan (2008) puts forward the case for midwives and obstetricians to abandon their stance and posturing, what he labels as 'professional positioning' and work more collaboratively to safeguard the wellbeing of mothers and babies. As great strides are made into the new Millennium he questions whether maternity care in the UK is truly woman-centred. Implying the dichotomy that currently exists between the social and medical model of care is unhelpful as it serves only to polarise views of pregnancy and childbirth, and does little to harmonise both professional groups. Pregnancy and childbirth, he argues, is a continuum and a very dynamic process where there are no absolutes especially in the context of risks. Each woman is an individual, some have complex psychosocial and physical needs that make them vulnerable, others seem to sail through the process without any difficulty. Categorising women 'pigeonholes' them and suggests a 'cache pot' even though one size does not fit all. What is important is to be flexible and adaptable in order to be responsive to women's needs.

Good team work and good outcomes for mothers and babies require positive and effective communication between midwife and doctors who need to relate as professional equals (Healthcare Commission (HC) 2006, 2008). It is vital to have unification not only between women and midwives but between midwives and the other members of the interprofessional team, especially obstetricians. There are compelling arguments to strengthen the autonomous role of the midwife and there are a number of socio-political drivers for change that have emerged from the Department of Health (DH 1993, 1998, 2001a, 2001b, 2001c, 2003a, 2003b, 2004, 2007, 2008a, 2008b) and have been useful in supporting change.

Conclusion

The midwife–mother relationship forms the backbone of midwifery care. Being pregnant and having a baby is not just about a safe biophysical outcome for the mother and baby. It embodies the social, psychological, emotional and spiritual dimensions of care. The journey relates to relationships and how the woman feels about herself, the care she receives from the midwife and her overall satisfaction with that experience. The emotional work involved in the whole experience for both the woman and midwife should not be underestimated. The very essence of a profound experience like pregnancy, birth and motherhood captures aspects of women's lives and define who they are as individuals. It also defines women's bodies, women's sexuality, women's power and the knowledge and wisdom women share. Understanding the psychological consequences of power and powerlessness is important as there is no place for power imbalance in maternity care. Disempowered midwives often mean disempowered women. Midwives who are powerless may act without direction in their attempt to influence change, only to have their efforts thwarted by those in power who may be fearful of losing their credibility and looking foolish.

Any working relationship between different professional groups needs time and effort on the part of all disciplines. Effective and collaborative teamwork will only materialise when there is understanding and mutual respect for professional boundaries. Coupled with this there also needs to be recognition of the skill, knowledge and expertise all members of the interprofessional team bring to such encounters. The complex organisation of care within the NHS means that midwives and doctors need to work to achieve cognisance of each other's role and respect the contribution each make to maternity care. A respectful and supportive partnership between allied professionals and a positive working environment will ensure that the care of mothers and babies is not compromised and there is good psychological outcome (HC 2006, 2008).

Finally, student midwives are the future hope of the midwifery profession. They need a solid and meaningful relationship with their mentors. The learning environment in which student midwives are socialised and educated should therefore be supportive of their emotional needs. This is necessary if they are to develop an understanding of the philosophy of woman-centred care, and acquire the toolkit of knowledge, skills, values and beliefs that are so essential to 'being with woman'.

Summary of key points

- Midwifery is an interactive profession and arguably the whole practice of midwifery and the ethos of being 'with woman' are non-existent without a relationship of trust.

- Trust binds midwives and women together.

- Women need to trust midwives to have confidence in their abilities and to protect and safeguard the foundations of normality.

- A modern NHS needs empowered midwives who can sculpt a woman-centred philosophy of care, support women in their choices and help bring a real shift in the balance of power.

- A respectful relationship instils confidence, ensures reciprocity and values the individual regardless of their socioeconomic status, socio-cultural background, sexual orientation, colour or ethnicity.

- Midwives' relationships should build solidarity. It is important to choose the correct language and behaviour when interacting with women.

- Students need positive role models and support from mentors to become autonomous practitioners who understand the 'with woman' philosophy.

References

Altman, I. and Taylor, D. (1973) *Social Penetration: The Development of Interpersonal Relationships.* New York: Holt, Rhinehart and Winston.

Ball, L., Curtis, P. and Kirkham, M. (2002) *Why Do Midwives Leave? The women's informed childbearing and health research group.* www.rcm.org.uk, accessed 4 June 2009.

Begley, C.M. (2001a) 'Knowing your place': student midwives' views on relationships in midwifery in Ireland. *Midwifery,* 17(3): 222–33.

Begley, C.M. (2001b) Giving midwifery care: student midwives' views of their working role. *Midwifery*, 17(1): 24–34.

Bick, D. (2008) Enhancing safety in maternity services: a greater role for midwife-led care? *Midwifery*, 25(1): 1–2.

Cameron, J. and Ellwood, D. (2006) Choices, collaboration and outcomes in Australia. In: A. Symon (ed.) *Risk and Choice in Maternity care: an international perspective*. Edinburgh: Churchill Livingstone, pp 139–48.

Cameron, J. and Taylor, J. (2007) Nursing and midwifery: re-evaluating the relationship. *International Journal of Nursing Studies*, 44: 855–6.

Curtis, P., Ball, L. and Kirkham, M. (2006) Bullying and horizontal violence: cultural or individual phenomena? *British Journal of Midwifery*, 14(4): 218–21.

Davies, R.M. and Atkinson, P. (1991) Students of midwifery: 'doing the obs' and other coping strategies. *Midwifery*, 7(3): 113–21.

Department of Health (2008a) *High Quality Care for All: NHS Next Stage Review Final Report* (Darzi Report). www.dh.gov.uk, accessed 1 June 2009.

Department of Health (2008b) *Framing the Nursing and Midwifery Contribution: Driving up the Quality of care*. www.dh.gov.uk, accessed 1 June 2009.

Department of Health (2007) *Maternity Matters: Access and Continuity of Care in a Safe Service*. www.dh.gov.uk, accessed 1 June 2009.

Department of Health (2004) *National Service Framework for Children, Young People and Maternity Services*. www.dh.gov.uk, accessed 1 June 2009.

Department of Health (2003a) *Modern Matrons – Improving Patient Experience*. www.dh.gov.uk, accessed 1 June 2009.

Department of Health (2003b) *Approval of Nurse, Midwife and Health Visitor Consultant Posts; PLCNO(2003)5*. www.dh.gov.uk, accessed 1 June 2009.

Department of Health (2001a) *Working Together, Learning Together: A framework for lifelong learning in the NHS*. www.dh.gov.uk, accessed 1 June 2009.

Department of Health (2001b) *Making a Difference: the nursing, midwifery and health visiting contribution – the midwifery action plan*. www.dh.gov.uk, accessed 1 June 2009.

Department of Health (2001c) *Shifting the Balance of Power within the NHS: securing delivery*. www.dh.gov.uk, accessed 1 June 2009.

Department of Health (1998) *European Working Time Directive*. www.dh.gov.uk, accessed 1 June 2009.

Department of Health (1993) *Hospital Doctors: Training for the Future* (Calman Report). www.dh.gov.uk, accessed 1 June 2009.

Dornan, J.C. (2008) Is childbirth in the UK really mother centred? *International Journal of Nursing Studies*, 45(6): 809–11.

Foucault, M. (2001) *Power. Volume 111: essential works of Foucault 1954–1984*. London: Penguin.

Freeman, L.M. (2006) Continuity of carer and partnership: a review of the literature. *Women and Birth*, 19 (2): 39–44.

Freire, P. (1993) *The Pedagogy of the Oppressed*, 2nd edn. London: Penguin.

Halldorsdottir, S. and Karlsdottir, S. (1996) Empowerment or discouragement: women's experience of caring and uncaring encounters during childbirth. *Health Care Women International*, 17: 361–79.

Hatem, M., Sandall, J., Devane, D., Soltani, H. and Gates, S. (2008) Midwife-led versus other models of care for childbearing women. *Cochrane Database of Systematic Reviews*. Art No: CD004667. DOI: 10.10021/14651858.

Healthcare Commission (2008) *Towards Better Births: a review of maternity services in England*. http://www.cqc.org.uk, accessed 12 June 2009.

Healthcare Commission (2006) *Investigation into 10 Maternal Deaths at, or Following Delivery at Northwick Park Hospital, Northwest London Hospitals NHS Trust between April 2002–April 2005*. http://www.cqc.org.uk, accessed 12 June 2009.

Hildebrand, J. and Markovic, D. (2007) Systemic therapists' experience of powerlessness. *Australian and New Zealand Journal of Family Therapy*, 28(4): 191–9, accessed online at www.atypon-link.com 1 July 2009.

Hunter, B. (2006) The importance of reciprocity in relationships between community based midwives and mothers. *Midwifery*, 22(4): 308–22.

Hunter, B. and Deery, R. (eds) (2009) *Emotions in Midwifery and Reproduction*. Basingstoke: Macmillan.

Hunter, L.P. (2008) A hermeneutic phenomenological analysis of midwives ways of knowing during childbirth. *Midwifery*, 24(4): 405–15.

Jones, C. and Wylie, L. (2008) An exploration of the factors that cause stress to student midwives in the clinical setting. *Midwives online:* www.rcm.org.uk, accessed 4 June 2009.

Kirkham, M. (2009) Emotion work around reproduction: supportive or constraining? In: B. Hunter, R. Deery (eds) *Emotions in Midwifery and Reproduction*. Basingstoke: Macmillan, pp 227–37.

Kirkham, M. (2007) *Traumatised Midwives*. www.aims.org.uk/Journal/Vol19No1/traumatisedMidwives.htm, accessed 1 June 2009.

Kirkham, M. (2003) Midwifery in the NHS (editorial). *Association of Radical Midwives*, www.radmid. demon.co.uk, accessed 1 July 2009.

Kirkham, M. (2000) How can we relate? In: M. Kirkham (ed.) *The Midwife–Woman Relationship*. Basingstoke: Palgrave Macmillan, pp 227–50.

Kirkham, M. (1999) The culture of midwifery in the NHS in England. *Journal of Advanced Nursing*, 30(3): 732–9.

Kirkham, M., Morgan, R.K. and Davies, A. (2006) *Why do Midwives Stay?* www.rcm.org.uk, accessed 4 June 2009.

Kirkham, M., Stapleton, H., Thomas, G. and Curtis, P. (2002) Checking not listening: how midwives cope. *British Journal of Midwifery*, 10(7): 447–50.

Lavender, T., Walkinshaw, S.A. and Walton, I. (1999) A prospective study of women's views of factors contributing to a positive birth experience. *Midwifery*, 15(1): 40–6.

Leap, N. (2000) The less we do, the more we give. In: M. Kirkham (ed.) *The Midwife–Woman Relationship*. Basingstoke: Palgrave Macmillan, pp 1–18.

Lundgren, I. and Berg, M. (2007) Central concepts in the midwife–woman relationship. *Scandinavian Journal of Caring Sciences*, 21(2): 220–8.

McCourt, C. and Stevens, T. (2009) Relationship and reciprocity in caseload midwifery. In: B. Hunter, R. Deery (eds) *Emotions in Midwifery and Reproduction*. Basingstoke: Macmillan, pp 17–35.

McCourt C, Page L, Hewison J, Vail A (1998) Evaluation of one-to-one midwifery: women's responses to care. *Birth*, 25:73–80.

National Institute for Health and Clinical Excellence (2008) *Antenatal Care: routine care for the healthy pregnant women, CG 62*. London: NICE. www.nice.org.uk, accessed 1 June 2009.

Nursing and Midwifery Council (2009) *Standards for Pre-registration Midwifery Education*. London: NMC.

Nursing and Midwifery Council (2004) *Midwives Rules and Standards*. London: NMC.

O'Neill, O. (2008) *Safe Births: Everybody's Business. An independent inquiry into safety of maternity services in England*. London: King's Fund.

Page, L. (2003) *One-to-one Midwifery Care: restoring the 'with woman' relationship in midwifery*. www.medscape.com, accessed 18 May 2009.

Pembroke, N.F. and Pembroke, J.J. (2006) The spirituality of presence in midwifery care. *Midwifery*, 24(3): 321–7.

Powell-Kennedy, H.P., Shannon, M.T. and Kravetz, M.K. (2004) The landscape of caring for women: a narrative study of midwifery practice. *Journal of Midwifery and Women's Health*, 49(1): 14–23.

Randle, J. (2006) *Workplace Bullying in the NHS*. Oxford: Radcliffe Press.

Sandall, J., Davies, J. and Warwick, C. (2001) *Evaluation of the Albany Midwifery Practice: Final Report*. London: Florence Nightingale School of Nursing and Midwifery, Kings College.

Siddiqui, J. (1999) The therapeutic relationship in midwifery. *British Journal of Midwifery*, 7(2): 111–14.

Smith, A.H., Dixon, A.L. and Page, L.A. (2009) Health-care professionals' views about safety in maternity services: a qualitative study. *Midwifery*, 25(1): 21–31.

Stapleton, H., Kirkham, M., Thomas, G. and Curtis, P. (2002a) Midwives in the middle: balance and vulnerability. *British Journal of Midwifery*, 10(10): 607–11.

Stapleton, H., Kirkham, M., Curtis, P. and Thomas, G. (2002b) Stereotyping as a professional defence mechanism. *British Journal of Midwifery*, 10(9): 549–52.

Thompson, F.E. (2005) The ethical nature of the mother–midwife relationship: a feminist perspective. *Australian Midwifery*, 18(3): 17–21.

Thornstensen, K.A. (2000) Trusting women: essential to midwifery. *Journal of Midwifery and Women's Health*, 45(5): 405–7.

Thornstensson, S., Nissen, E. and Ekström, A. (2008) An exploration and description of student midwives experiences in offering continuous labour support to women/couples. *Midwifery*, 24(4): 451–9.

Walsh, D. (2006) 'Nesting' and 'matrescence' as destructive features of a free-standing birth centre in the UK. *Midwifery*, 22(3): 228–39.

Yearsley, C. (1999) Pre-registration student midwives: fitting in. *British Journal of Midwifery*, 7(10): 627–31.

Annotated further reading

Fahy, K., Foureur, M. and Hastie, C. (eds) (2008) *Birth Territory and Midwifery Guardianship: theory for practice, education and research*. London: Elsevier.

This text provides a pragmatic approach and thought provoking ideas for midwives and women to maintain guardianship of normality during childbirth.

Green, J.M., Bastion, H., Easton, S. and McCormick, F. (2003) *Greater expectations? Inter-relationships between women's expectations and experiences of decision making, continuity, choice and control in labour, and psychological outcomes: summary report*. University of Leeds: Mother and Infant Research Unit.

The title speaks for itself.

Lundgren, I. (2004) Releasing and relieving encounters: experiences of pregnancy and childbirth. *Scandinavian Journal of Caring Sciences*, 18(4): 368–75.

Highlights the importance of creating positive memories for women as the encounters they have with midwives may remain indelibly imprinted in their minds.

3 Emotions during pregnancy, labour and puerperium

Chapter contents

Introduction

Chapter aims

The link between the social and psychological
dimensions of pregnancy, labour and the
puerperium

Transitional crises

Motherhood

Fatherhood

Normative adjustment reactions during
pregnancy, labour and the puerperium

Conclusion

Summary of key points

References

Annotated further reading

Useful websites

Introduction

Pregnancy, labour and the puerperium are periods in a woman's life which are often associated with the full range of human emotions, not dissimilar to those apparent in other major life events or life transitions. Assessment of psychological health is therefore an integral part of the midwife's role as she is charged with having key responsibility in promoting health and wellbeing for childbearing women (International Confederation of Midwives (ICM) 2005, NMC 2004). Equally she should be vigilant in recognising and detecting early any deviation from the normative responses commonly experienced as part of the parenting role. The distinction between what is perceived as normative psychological adjustment reactions and those associated with pathological changes as delineated in Chapter 4, is important in order to avoid unnecessary medicalisation of women's moods. Moreover, the midwife has responsibility for helping to foster confidence in women and their partners, and support these couples in developing and nurturing healthy parent–baby relationships (Chapter 9). Midwives who have insight and understanding of the diverse psychological factors that can influence feelings, emotions, thoughts and behaviours during the pregnancy continuum, are well placed in meeting the needs of women and their partners. This chapter is an attempt to explore some of the issues of importance to women's psychological health and wellbeing during pregnancy, labour and the puerperium. There is also general acknowledgement that the emotional reactions that may arise during these transitional phases are as important as the physical ones.

> **Chapter aims**
>
> - To examine the range of diverse but common human emotions that may affect women during pregnancy, labour and the puerperium
> - To highlight the relevance of body image to psychological health
> - To discuss the myths and ideology surrounding parenthood in order to reflect on it as a maturational crisis in the lives of mothers and fathers
> - To explore how the arrival of a new baby impacts on relationships, roles and family dynamics
> - To consider issues of diversity and factors that can make women psychologically vulnerable
> - To identify the midwife's role in supporting mothers and their partner throughout the pregnancy continuum

The link between the social and psychological dimensions of pregnancy, labour and the puerperium

Body image

The female body during pregnancy is a highly visible time for women and a period of significant change and contested meanings. Pregnancy for many women captures the essence of their womanhood and confers evidence of their femininity. It is influenced by cultural norms and social expectations, and imbued in stereotypes where the woman will either be revered or shunned. Representation of the female body at this time in psychological terms presents a dichotomy. On one hand women either adore being pregnant or feel at odds with their pregnant bodies. There are also those in the middle who may feel happy or ambivalent about their body image during pregnancy. This in part will be influenced by the different dimensions that influence a woman's view of herself such as **body image**, **self-esteem**, **self-concept**, **self-image** and **self-efficacy** (see Chapter 7). Society's relentless obsession with thinness contributes to how women view and judge themselves. Having a healthy body image means women feel comfortable in their own skin and accepting of who they are, and have the self-confidence to resist any pressure to conform to someone else's ideal or standard of 'perfection'. In order to develop an understanding of how psychology contributes to an understanding of body image, readers are invited to complete the questions outlined in the quiz detailed in Box 3.1.

Box 3.1 Quiz: Does your body image affect you? Circle *yes* or *no* to indicate the most appropriate response that best apply to you.

Do you regularly calculate your **body mass index** (BMI)?	Yes/No
Is your BMI between 20 and 25?	Yes/No
Are you concerned by your BMI or does it affect the way you feel about yourself?	Yes/No
Do you weigh yourself frequently?	Yes/No
Is the idea of being lean and well toned just a matter of personal discipline?	Yes/No

Do you have an ideal body weight?	Yes/No
Do you ever skip meals in order to lose weight?	Yes/No
Would your **self-image** or **self-esteem** improve if you were to lose weight?	Yes/No
Do you experience feelings of guilt after eating a full meal?	Yes/No
When you are feeling sad, do you use food as a comfort measure?	Yes/No
In terms of body image and attractiveness are you influenced by images of slim women/men as depicted in the popular media (e.g. women's/men's magazines, newspaper, television, billboards etc)?	Yes/No
Are you influenced by the messages that surround you in how you should look or dress?	Yes/No
Do you recognise or have resisted negative media influences?	Yes/No
Are media images of female sexuality/standard of beauty limited in their representations?	Yes/No

The pressure to achieve 'perfection' in appearance through weight is intense. If readers answered 'yes' to all or some of the questions in the quiz, such responses would mirror those of the general population and indeed pregnant women. Limited research has examined women's image of their bodies during pregnancy and their attitudes and behaviour to the inherent changes. A study by Skouters et al (2005) found that psychosocial factors contribute to body image changes in pregnancy. Women studied experienced higher levels of dissatisfaction with their body image in early to mid second trimester than in the third trimester of pregnancy, but felt less attractive in late pregnancy though not necessarily dissatisfied with their body image. However, Boscaglia et al (2003) report that body image was fairly stable in pregnancy, and women were able to adjust to the bodily changes of pregnancy without any negative connotations. This would suggest that women who became pregnant harbouring concerns about their body image will tend to maintain them and vice versa. Social psychology would also indicate that generally women who are physically fit and continue to embrace exercise during pregnancy as part of their lifestyle, may possibly respond more favourably to changes in their bodies compared to women who remain sedentary during pregnancy.

Influence of the media

The media plays an important role in Western society on how body image and female sexuality are engendered. Media image of perfection tends to relate to women who are young, thin and white, culminating in a narrow definition and standard of beauty. Women from minority ethnic groups, older women, women with disability and fat women are often missing from the picture and are somewhat 'symbolically annihilated' and marginalised (Barnes and Balber 2007). Paradoxically, these women, not subjected to the **panoptical** or microscopic gaze of the media in the same way, are much freer to express their sexuality. Yet this group of women deviate from the 'norm' and ultimately are not as objectified in the same way as the more dominant images of female beauty. Grabe et al (2008) suggest that media images of 'perfection' or idealised bodies only serve to objectify and sexualise women, culminating in body image concerns for women with profound psychological implications that can lead to depression. Midwives should acknowledge how a woman's body image may affect the way she feels about herself as a woman, and consider the implications of these feelings on the woman's moods as well as her adjustment to motherhood.

Obesity versus thinness

Schwartz and Brownell (2004) assert that modern Western society denigrates large women and emphasises thinness to the extent that women who have a **body mass index** (BMI) over 35 experience stigma and stereotypical attitudes in their day-to-day life. The health benefits of not being anorexic or obese are widely acknowledged World Health Organization (WHO 2004), and it is best for women and men to plan pregnancy after achieving optimal health. However, with the growing celebrity culture and a burgeoning obesity crisis, pregnancy is a time of changing attitudes toward the female body where perceptions have been altered. In recent years numerous celebrities have been captured displaying their pregnant bellies with great pride and much aplomb. The media fails to identify that weight gain in pregnancy is part of the normal biophysical changes women's bodies have to make to adapt physiologically to pregnancy. In Western culture it almost seems to be a conspiracy with the tyrannical way in which the media bombards popular culture with images of skinny women. This puts further pressure on mothers by perpetuating the myth of new mothers in the celebrity world losing their post-baby weight with breakneck speed to regain their pre-pregnancy figure. It is easy for women to fall prey to such media fodder and irresponsible reporting if their body image is already threatened (Boscaglia et al 2003). It would appear that postpartum is the period when women are most unhappy with their bodies (Skouters et al 2005). Women are raised to view their bodies as a means of achieving control; therefore, body image and self-esteem are inextricably linked, which may be mirrored in women's attitude and behaviour during pregnancy, childbirth and beyond. Such knowledge can be helpful to midwives in listening and attending to women as it will influence how they communicate and support women during these periods.

There are other psychosocial issues that affect a woman's body image and whether a woman is thin or obese. Maio et al (2006) outline a number of salient points that are of relevance to midwifery practice, such as the role of ambivalence in promoting and aiding the individual to adopt healthy behaviours. Emphasis on public health information on what foods to avoid, it is argued, misses the point somewhat where deeply rooted feelings of ambivalence prevails. A literature review conducted by Foresight (2007) outlines the negative correlation between obesity, education, socio-economic status and mental health. Obesity can lead not only to a negative body image but it can make the woman vulnerable in other ways. Misguided prejudice and discrimination can result in stereotypical attitudes or indeed social exclusion where the woman is disenfranchised and may receive care that is both ineffective and insensitive. Foresight (2007) suggests that obesity is more evident in the poorer sections of society. The notion of ambivalence as a psychological concept and a health issue, serves as a useful reminder that obesity and thinness are very complex psychological and social issues that may be linked to social class and social divide. Although the extremes of weight are more intricate than the matter of body image can realistically provide an explanation for, there is little doubt that they cause physical and psychological morbidity. Figure 3.1 summarises some of the factors that may affect body image.

Transitional crises

Adjustment to change: role conflict

The transition to parenthood is heralded as a unique experience for women as well as men (Woolett and Parr 1997). Gross and Pattison (2007), Callister (1996) and Jordan (1980) provide a cross-cultural perspective of pregnancy, childbirth and parenthood. This assists in the understanding that regardless of culture and society, the transition to parenthood is a ceremonial rite of passage, and one of the most exciting and testing moments for women and men. It

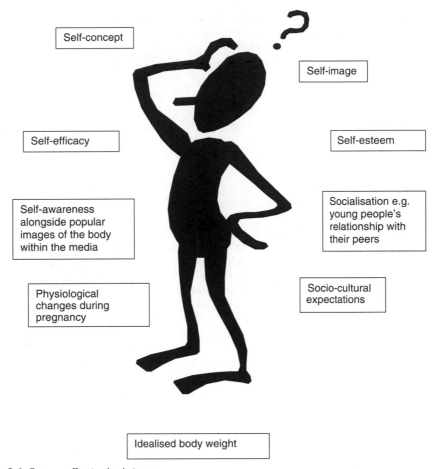

Figure 3.1 Factors affecting body image

commences with the realisation of pregnancy and the climax of birth, bringing about marked changes within the couple's relationship, family dynamics and friendships. It is also a time of individual fulfilment, joy and contentment. If it is the first baby, it signifies changes to the relationship for the couple from a dyad to a triad. Roles and responsibilities shift with the possibility of such alterations affecting employment, finances, relocation, and the couple's co-dependence on each other or desire to cling onto their independence. This may result in stress, anxiety, conflict and tension. The reader is invited to review the case vignette outlined in Case scenario 3.1 and identify the possible sources of conflict in Sophie's and Sam's relationship.

Case scenario 3.1

Sophie is 19 years old, 37 weeks pregnant with her first baby. She lives with her partner Sam, who is 28 years old and a manager at their local supermarket. The pregnancy is unplanned but the couple are both excited by the prospect of becoming parents. They live in rented accommodation. Sophie is studying to be a nursery nurse. The couple have no immediate family living nearby but have a close circle of friends. Sophie wants to relocate where they can be nearer to their respective families as the baby will be the first grandchild for their parents. Sam has developed a close network of friends and is less keen on the idea.

Reflective activity

1. What are the most striking issues arising from this case vignette that you think are likely to have the greatest psychological impact?
2. From a psychological perspective how might the pregnancy affect Sophie and Sam's relationship?

Having a baby is a time when a couple like Sophie and Sam are most likely to relocate in order to have better housing be it in the private or public sector, adding to further stressors. Although some relationships improve during this period of adjustment and change, others will deteriorate. Sophie and Sam will find that pregnancy and birth place huge demands on them as parents and put a major degree of stress and strain on their relationship, as their roles and responsibilities alter. This could strengthen their relationship and bring them closer together. Equally, such a profound change could put a wedge between them and act as the catalyst for the demise of their partnership, especially if the bonds cementing it were already fragile. There is a higher incidence of relationship breakdown during the period of early parenthood as children do not necessarily bring happiness to a relationship (Powdhavee 2009, Gilbert 2006). The arrival of a new baby not only amounts to a major shift in the couple's relationship, but it also raises challenges in terms of the couple's social network. The challenges imposed are not necessarily negative as the couple might seize them as opportunities to grow, develop and learn together during their journey into parenthood.

Raynor (2006) highlights that friendships, particularly those of the mother, will be tested, for example social expectations and the degree of social support such networks can and do provide. It is likely that old acquaintances, especially friends who have no children of their own, may be weakened. Some relationships can either be strengthened or even replaced gradually by new contacts established through forging relationships with other parents, developed during parent education classes or postnatal mother and baby support groups. Changes also occur with the relationship with other family members. The new parents will find that their parents now have to develop roles as grandparents. If the couple have existing children, these children may feel slightly pushed out and find that they are competing for attention from their parents with the addition of the new baby. The couple too have to undergo role changes on an individual level as well as accepting their parenting role. No longer are they just a daughter or son, they have become a mother and father. Role conflict and confusion are often the reality due to the competing demands on their time of caring for a new baby and performing other roles in their daily lives. Mothers may find that there is little time for them to pursue other activities, which can diminish any opportunity for contact with and support from others. This is particularly the case if they have an unsupported partner, are socially isolated and indeed if they have had twins or higher multiples. Psychological care during the postnatal period should therefore take account of the social factors that can affect women's emotional wellbeing e.g. quality of support, poverty and number of small children in the household (National Institute for Health and Clinical Excellence (NICE) 2006, DH 2004).

Pregnancy usually means that if the woman is employed she will have to cease employment at some stage to commence maternity leave. Some women give up work altogether while others who return will either do so full time or may resume employment in a totally different capacity. Some may even job share or change their contract to work on a part-time basis. The role of the partner may also change, depending on who is the main breadwinner within the household. Some men take on the role as house husband if they earn less than their partner and the couple agree that this is the most viable and sensible solution in embracing partnership in their role as parents, and dealing with their economic situation.

Motherhood

Motherhood as a maturational crisis: myths and ideology

In order to think about motherhood and fatherhood as socially constructed terms the reader is invited to complete the questions in Box 3.2.

Box 3.2 Reflective activity: social construction of motherhood and fatherhood

1. What do you understand by the terms motherhood and fatherhood?
2. Are these terms biologically determined or influenced by culture, socio-economic and political factors?
3. What factors influence the maternal and paternal role?
4. What are the stereotypical roles ascribed to mothers and fathers?
5. What are the characteristics that define whether a woman/man is perceived as a 'good' or 'bad' parent?
6. How can midwives support parents to experience a positive transition to their parenting role?

Motherhood is an essential feature of women's lives, and one of the few universal roles allotted to women, despite there being no universal experience of motherhood as outlined by O'Reilly (2004: 5): '. . . motherhood is primarily not a natural function; rather, it is specifically and fundamentally a cultural practice that is continuously redesigned in response to changing economic and societal factors. As a cultural construct, its meaning varies with time and place; there is no essential or universal experience of motherhood.'

Motherhood and fatherhood are not biologically determined roles; they are influenced and defined by social constructs, culture, socio-economic factors and politics. However, regardless of the view of a more supposedly liberated and permissive society, gender role and biases still exist in the context of parenthood. The views towards the role of men and women in Western societies regarding childrearing have not altered significantly with generational changes. The fact remains that when it comes to childcare, mothers are still the main care-giver. It is also a stark fact that it is women who bear much of the responsibility in managing the home. However, women's angst, rage and general feelings of dissatisfaction with their role of mother and lover may stem from poor support from their partner rather than the role per se, and is a root cause of unhappiness in women's lives (Grabowska 2009, Oakley et al 1996).

Motherhood is full of dichotomies, paradoxes or contradictions as it can be the toughest, most demanding, challenging and yet the most fulfilling, satisfying and rewarding of life experiences. Some feminists have taken issue with how motherhood is depicted and por-trayed in society (Nicholson 1997). Furthermore, O'Reilly (2004, 2008) argues that the term motherhood is limited as it is socially constructed within patriarchal structures rendering it oppressive to women. Mothering, she argues, is a more empowering concept for women as it acknowledges women's experiences, not only as mothers but as women. These experiences for women she emphasises are a rich source of female power. Being a 'good enough' parent requires patience, commitment, flexibility, resilience and an ability to respond, not only to the baby's physical needs, but also to the infant's developmental needs on an emotional, social, behavioural and cognitive level. Therefore, parents must learn what constitutes normative behavioural patterns at each stage of the baby's growth and development (see Chapter 9).

'Good' versus 'bad' mother debate

The notion of motherhood is a shared experience among women in both Western and more traditional cultures, in that motherhood is still governed by patriarchal structures, even though these women's lives are diametrically opposed. Women in Western cultures, unlike some women in more traditional societies, tend to have access to contraception and can exercise their reproductive rights to make decisions and exercise choice and control over their reproductive health in terms of family planning and spacing. The term motherhood is, therefore, seen as problematic for women on a number of counts. It is a time when women are revered, as they fulfil their biological destiny, confirm their femininity and for some, raise their status in society, albeit without any financial gain. At the same time women may find that they are being judged as a 'good' or 'bad' mother (Winson 2009, Choi et al 2005, Silva 1996) as they grieve for the loss of their identity, their former life and struggle to feel fulfilled and satisfied with their mothering role. Some of the dichotomies posed by the notion of the 'good' and 'bad' mother are noted in the questions raised in Box 3.3. The reader is invited to reflect on these questions and think of their relevance to practice.

Box 3.3 Reflective activity

Who belongs to the 'good' mother vs the 'bad' mother club?

- Working vs stay at home mother?
- Lesbian vs heterosexual mother?
- Disabled vs able bodied mother?
- Teenage vs older mother?
- Single vs married mother?
- Mother from white middle class/dominant ethnic group vs mother who is non-white and from minority ethnic group?

Fatherhood

Ideology of fatherhood

Parallel to the discussion of motherhood is the myth of fatherhood, a social construct. Men's own experience of being fathered during childhood, how they live their lives and how the process of their socialisation helped to form their identities, will contribute to how they develop and foster relationships within their family structure. The way in which men are parented is important whether this experience mirrors difficult or positive issues.

'Good' and 'bad' dads

Like motherhood, two contrasting images of fathers prevail that have been created by the media and reflected as a dichotomy and emerging theme in the literature as illustrated in Box 3.4.

Box 3.4 'Good' vs 'bad' father as a social construct

Features of the 'good' father	Features of the 'bad' father
middle-class	socio-economically deprived
loving, stable family-oriented	emotionally detached or challenged
employed and hardworking	unemployed and lazy
contribute to their child's security, care and wellbeing, emotionally, socially, financially and psychologically	promiscuous, 'a bit of a lad' persona largely deviant, absent or marginally involved
Good role model	Poor role model

The media's representation of the 'missing dad' or fathers who play a marginal role in their children's life is all too common. Yet the majority of men play an active part in their children's upbringing. Children benefit from a sound relationship with their fathers. Preliminary results released by a report *Growing up with Dad* from Children in Wales and the young people's charity Catch 22 (www.catch22.org.uk) have demonstrated that children who enjoy an enduring and good relationship with their fathers are less likely to engage in anti-social behaviour, abuse alcohol, take illicit drugs, or smoke. The figures identified in Table 3.1 are part of the analysis of the survey undertaken by Catch 22 (2009) of almost 18,000 young people across Wales. This was initiated as part of the *Communities that Care* programme. This analysis resonates with the emerging body of evidence that a healthy father–child relationship is instrumental to the socialisation and cognitive development of children.

Table 3.1 Result of Catch 22 (2009) Survey

	(Number involved in survey 18,000)
Children living with their father who feel close to him	86%
Children not living with their father who still feel close to him	47%
Boys who feel close to their father	79%
Girls who feel close to their father	69%
15-year-olds who have tried cannabis	28%
15-year-olds close to their father who had tried cannabis	24%
15-year-olds not close to their father who had tried cannabis	39%

Source: **Growing up with Dad.** Catch22: www.catch22.org.uk

Young fathers and the 'Dad Deficit'

The Fatherhood Institute (2008) published a report that highlights research calling for health-care professionals to engage more with fathers, especially those who are young, during the maternity period to ensure that their needs are met. The main recommendations from this report of importance to midwifery practice that will ensure greater involvement of fathers are summarised in Box 3.5.

Box 3.5 The Fatherhood Institute (2008) recommendations to address the 'dad deficit'

Acknowledgement of the importance of birth registration for fathers: 45,000 men in the UK do not sign the birth certificate when their child is born (equivalent to 7% of all births – and double the rate in Australia).

NHS guidance on father-inclusion is needed such as more family friendly environment within the hospital setting. When surveyed the majority of men and women agree that dads should be able to stay overnight in hospital with their partner when the baby is born as some men literally felt 'shut out' when visiting hours is over. It is reported that 86% of fathers attend the birth of their child.

Information for fathers explaining their role in smoking, breastfeeding, alcohol, mental health and baby health is needed.

Dealing with relationship stress and conflict and the impact of violence in the family needs further prominence.

Preconception-education of fathers stressing the importance of optimal health when planning a family.

Midwives supporting men as fathers

A literature review conducted by Plantin (2007a) revealed an affirmative approach: involvement by fathers not only results in positive health effects for them but also contributes to the psychological, social and physical wellbeing of their children and partner. Additionally it has been shown that men can be a source of psychological strength and support to women throughout the maternity context (Oakley et al 1996). Midwives have a pivotal part to play by engaging with men and providing appropriate parent education sessions to meet their needs. Research reported by the Department of Health (DH 2008a, 2008b) reveals that despite the positive influence that men can have on the family unit, there is a yawning gap between the support afforded to women and men during the antenatal period to aid their adjustment and transition to parenthood. Plantin (2007a) highlights this as a good example of men feeling marginalised through the difficulty experienced in accessing and being involved in parent education classes specifically related to their needs. Young fathers in particular are identified as a group that the maternity service needs to target. The DH (2008a) revealed that 1:15 of all births in England are to young women under 20 years old; this group were responsible for approximately 45,000 births in 2006. Neglecting the needs of fathers perpetuates gender inequalities, and the continuation of custom and tradition relating to the social divide between men and women in assuming responsibility for paid employment and childcare. Plantin (2007b) also asserts that the infrastructure should support fathers being more visible on the agenda of policy makers, service providers and the healthcare professionals like midwives responsible for the delivery of care. Since traditional parent education classes disadvantage men, Plantin (2007a) suggests a more varied and innovative approach is needed such as internet sources and facilities to provide support on an individual basis. When setting up services aimed at meeting the needs of men, midwives must consider cultural taboos and expectations, factors influencing men's identity and masculinity as well as the multi-faceted aspects of support. Plantin (2007b) cites exemplars of good practice such as the Scandinavian example where fathers are generously supported by legislation regarding paternity leave and pay. This provides a good example of where culture, politics and legislation work harmoniously together to ensure there is a framework in place to support family friendly work environment and subsidised childcare facilities. Fathers, like mothers, are not a homogeneous group: the approach to education and skills training in readiness for parenthood offered by midwives should be eclectic in its approach. Midwives need to build a critical mass of evidence on how to best meet the needs of a diverse population, especially those with known vulnerability factors represented in Figure 3.2.

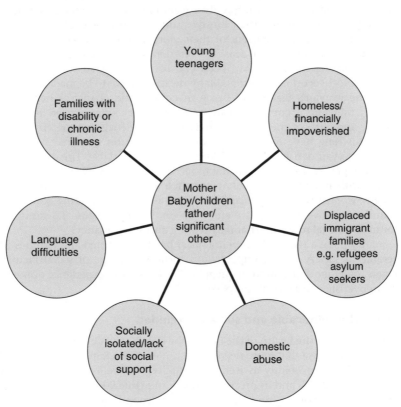

Figure 3.2 Vulnerability factors relating to social adversity that have implications for psychological health/ wellbeing

An understanding of gender roles and how these are learned and shaped in early life are important. However, the midwife should be mindful that these roles are different throughout cultures and both sexes, which can lead to inequality amongst both girls and boys and influence later experiences of both women/men and mothers/fathers. The midwife response should be threefold:

- to build evidence and take key steps in understanding and meeting the needs of both expectant mothers and fathers
- to work collaboratively with community groups and outside agencies to ensure inclusion of factors that will aid the development of strategies and resources to meet individual needs
- to develop a supporting role to advance not only the rights of fathers but also to protect the rights of mothers and prevent gender inequality.

Normative adjustment reactions during pregnancy, labour and the puerperium

Pregnancy

Pregnancy signifies a time of enormous change socially, biophysically and psychologically. It is a cultural phenomenon that denotes diverse emotions for all women. For most, the experience is a testing time as they alter their lifestyle and adjust to the challenges and demands of the pregnancy, and make preparation for their mothering role. Mood changes, fluctuations and disturbances at this time are at least as common as they are postpartum (Evans et al 2001). Symptoms relating to mood have been consistently associated with social factors, such as support and socio-economic factors. Many decisions have to be made which can be an ordeal and test the woman's feelings of being in control and challenge her coping mechanisms. Anxiety is therefore a common feature of pregnancy often linked to concerns about the pregnancy and birth of the baby. There is strong evidence that maternal anxiety and undue stress at this time have major implications not only on maternal wellbeing but also fetal development (Van den Bergh et al 2005, Teixeira et al 1999). This issue is explored in more detail in Chapter 7. However, it is vital to recognise that low mood and maternal unhappiness correlates with health abusive behaviour such as smoking. The reality for the most part is that many women will experience fluctuations of mood oscillating between ambivalence on one hand to positive and negative emotions on the other. Figure 3.3 summarises some of the common emotional reactions that may feature during pregnancy.

Pregnancy poses a risk to the psychological health of women and families who are the most vulnerable in society. This group account for a wide range of social factors such as young teenagers, older mothers, multiple pregnancies, those who experience domestic abuse and the most impoverished individuals in society.

Needs of the vulnerable and socially excluded

In order to improve the health of the nation the DH (2007a) developed a powerful public health message to emphasise that more needs to be done to help families who face social adversity to reduce the risk of morbidity as well as mortality. This report along with key findings from CEMACH (Lewis 2007) and its precursor (Lewis and Drife 2004) raises some thought-provoking issues. In the UK, women from the poorest backgrounds are 20 times more likely to die of a pregnancy related condition compared to those who are more affluent. Women who are severely disadvantaged are notoriously late bookers, accounting for 30% of late booking i.e. not presenting for maternity care until they are 20 weeks or more pregnant. If and when they do engage with services they often default, failing to keep their antenatal appointments. Women from minority ethnic groups, especially where English is not spoken as a first language, are also vulnerable; on average these women are three times more likely to die.

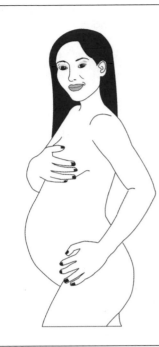

- pleasure, excitement, elation;
- dismay, disappointment, ambivalence;
- emotionally labile (e.g. episodes of weepiness exacerbated by physiological events such as nausea, vomiting and tiredness);
- psychological effects from physiological discomforts such as breast tenderness, backache and heartburn;
- increased femininity and a feeling of well-being especially as physiological effects of tiredness, or associated nausea and vomiting start to subside;
- a sense of increased attachment to the fetus; the impact of ultrasound scanning generating images for the prospective parents may intensify the experience;
- stress and anxiety about antenatal screening and diagnostic tests;
- increased demand for knowledge, information and need to make preparations for the birth accompanied by feelings of the need for increased detachment from work commitments;
- loss of or increased libido and altered body image;
- anxiety about labour (e.g. pain);
- anxiety about fetal abnormality, which may cause sleep disturbances/nightmares;
- increased vulnerability to major life events such as financial status, moving house, bereavement, or lack of a supportive partner.

Figure 3.3 Normative adjustment reactions during pregnancy

Domestic abuse

Domestic abuse is a major psychological issue of key public health concern within the UK as reported by DH (2005), Home Office for England (2008), Povey (2008) and the CEMACH report *Saving Mothers' Lives* (Lewis 2007). Emotionally and socially, women are affected on all levels as it occurs across society regardless of race, ethnicity, gender, age, wealth and country (Home Office 2008). It takes different forms from physical violence and psychological torture, to enforced marriages and female genital mutilation also known as honour violence (DH 2005). Box 3.6 identifies some stark statistics that although men are also affected by domestic abuse the odds are firmly stacked against women as detailed in the evidence by Povey (2008) and the Home Office (2008).

Box 3.6 Domestic Abuse: Significant Statistical Data (Povey 2008, Home Office 2008)

- Pregnancy and the early postnatal period are precursors to domestic abuse. Approximately 30% of domestic abuse begins during pregnancy or after childbirth and escalates during this time.
- 85% of reported incidents of domestic abuse the abused were women.
- 68% of women who experience domestic abuse knew the perpetrator and of these 65% were killed by their partner or ex-partner. This is in direct contrast to men where 44% of males who were abused knew the main and only suspect (11% killed by their partner or ex-partner).
- 83% of female victims of homicide were committed by partner/ex-partner 2006/07.
- 33% of violent incidents against women were domestic abuse, compared to 4% against men.
- Domestic abuse is implicated in 1:6 violent incidents.

- Domestic abuse is the only category of violence for which the risk is significantly elevated for women in comparison to men. This is despite a 65% fall in such incidents being reported since 1995.
- Repeated victimisation accounts for 75% of incidents with > 1:4 (27%) of sufferers experiencing repeated attacks 3–4 times or more.

Antenatal screening for domestic abuse

During the antenatal period it is imperative that midwives have the education and skills to make routine and sensitive enquiry about domestic abuse (Lewis 2007, DH 2005). Effective strategies must be in place such as multi-agency working, to ensure support and information is readily available to women at an early stage (DH 2004). Domestic abuse causes not only physical insults but damages the psychological and emotional wellbeing of women, destabilises the family and threatens the health of children on a very substantial scale.

Older mothers

The optimal biological age to have a baby is widely reported as 20 to 35 years old as the chance of conception is higher and the risks of morbidity reduced (WHO 2009). However, given that recent figures from the Office of National Statistics (ONS 2008) have shown a steep increase in pregnancies among the over-40s, more so than any other age group, the question of how old is too old to become a mother is omnipresent. It is reported that 1 in 7 couples are infertile (Bewley et al 2009) and fertility is affected by ageing; therefore, older women and their partners are more likely to be engaged in an emotional roller coaster in conceiving a baby. However, age remains a vexed subject that introduces double standards and a gender divide. It seems unfair to demonise older women as unselfish risk takers. The World Health Organization (WHO 2009) states that it is iniquitous to lay the blame for age related fertility problems squarely on the shoulders of women since having babies also involves men. Moreover, the psychology of being an older mother is not clearly understood, so to ascribe infertility to psychological factors, it is suggested, risks misattributing responsibility or victim blaming women. Age is only one factor of a multi-factorial and multi-complex issue. Ageing and reproductive ageing affect not only men and women as individuals but society as a whole. Addressing the double standard in this polemic highlights the stereotypical and divergent attitudes to men and women in society.

Multiple pregnancy

There is evidence that multiple pregnancy puts women at an elevated risk of psychological morbidity, which can jeopardise their mental health and wellbeing. This can manifest as complex grief reactions, stress, anxiety and depressive illness. The emotional impact of twin pregnancy and higher order multiple gestation is therefore an important issue for midwifery practice, especially with the increasing use of assisted means of reproduction such as in vitro fertilisation (IVF) in older women. Statistics from the ONS (2008) reveal that the trend in multiple births has doubled in the UK in comparison to 30 years ago. This increase is directly attributed to the growth in assisted reproduction techniques. Approximately 1 in 4 births result in twins or higher order multiples following IVF treatment. This figure is almost ten times higher than pregnancies that are naturally conceived, despite the strict controls imposed by the Human Fertilisation and Embryology Authority (HFEA 2008). Although such assisted means of reproduction provide tremendous benefits to women and their partners saddled with years of infertility problems, the psychological sequelae and medical risks associated with multiple pregnancy, birth and just being an older parent cannot be ignored. Whilst anxiety about the health and wellbeing of the developing fetus is a common experience in all pregnancies, this is doubled with multiple gestations, and is likely to be compounded if the parents are older.

The diagnosis of a multiple pregnancy can come as a real shock as it is often unexpected, especially with natural conceptions where there is no family history of multiple gestations. Such news might be greeted with joy and relief to utter anxiety and dismay. On the other hand, older women with an IVF multiple pregnancy might idealise the pregnancy, imagining that they will have their much longed for 'instant family' – the 'precious baby syndrome'. Evans et al (2001) report that the reassuring presence of the partner and empathetic approach of healthcare professionals who can communicate the diagnosis sensitively, can make a significant difference in the initial adjustment.

There is a higher risk of pregnancy complications for mother, fetus and neonate associated with multiple gestation compared to singleton pregnancies. These include miscarriage, fetal anomaly, preterm birth, low birth weight, caesarean section, stillbirth, intrauterine fetal death, pre-eclampsia, gestational diabetes, polyhydramnios, twin-to-twin transfusion (monozygotic twins), antepartum haemorrhage and other related maternal and perinatal morbidity. Such issues give even more cause for concern if the woman is older (Huang et al 2008, Hoffman et al 2007). However, Huang et al (2008) warn that maternal age alone is not a good discriminator for fetal/neonatal outcome. These factors all have emotional significance; prematurity for example results in low birth weight babies that may necessitate neonatal intensive care and a lengthy period of hospitalisation. This will involve protracted separation of the mother from her babies at birth, thus increasing maternal anxiety (Bryan 2003).

Antenatally, the woman might have concerns about her body image as her uterus expands and grows at an alarming rate. The physical morbidity associated with pregnancy such as nausea and vomiting, backache, oedema, and **striae gravidarum** can affect the way the woman feels about herself. As the pregnancy advances the woman might find that she tires easily and her mobility and positioning, especially for sleep, becomes difficult. She may no longer feel attractive or worry that her partner does not find her sexually attractive. Some men worry that coitus during pregnancy might be harmful; antenatal preparation classes should account for men's needs. Understandably if the couple have waited years to become parents and have undergone the rigours of IVF treatment they will be anxious and frightened about a possible pregnancy loss. Thus, what is perceived as minor ailments in pregnancy by midwives, might be a cause of great worry and concern for women.

Labour

The importance of the psychological and social dimensions of care during labour are well documented, which has been used to inform a plethora of reports and guidelines (Department of Health 2007b, 2004, NICE 2007, Redshaw et al 2007). Midwives as the guardians of normality should be able to facilitate choice for women by informing, supporting and helping them to feel in control of their labour and birth. The survey conducted by Redshaw et al (2007) found that women's perception of control during labour was influenced by four key factors: continuity of care with carer, one-to-one care in labour, not being left for long periods and being involved in decision-making. The philosophy of care during labour should, therefore, consider the common normative emotional responses at this time (see Figure 3.4) and the impact of the whole process on the woman's psychological health and wellbeing. Her experience should be one where positive memories are created, where her individuality and uniqueness are respected and where the potential for empowerment is transparent. This means the midwife has to work in such a manner that minimises disturbance, direction, intervention and meddlesomeness. The balance of power should be shifted towards the woman where the power of the woman to birth her baby is paramount. To achieve this woman-centred approach to care, midwives need

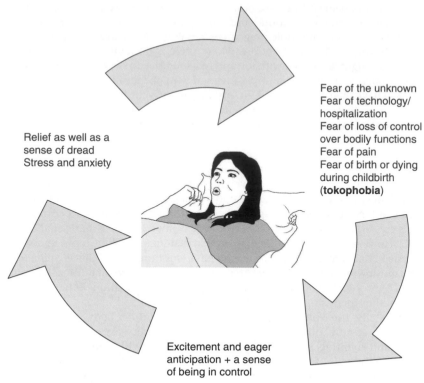

Fear of the unknown
Fear of technology/
hospitalization
Fear of loss of control
over bodily functions
Fear of pain
Fear of birth or dying
during childbirth
(**tokophobia**)

Relief as well as a
sense of dread
Stress and anxiety

Excitement and eager
anticipation + a sense
of being in control

Figure 3.4 Normative emotional responses to labour (Raynor 2006)

confidence and support to work in partnership with women, and to protect the dignity and privacy of birth.

The puerperium

Emotional responses during the puerperium are varied and contradictory. This is a pivotal period from birth to 6–8 weeks postpartum, when the woman is readjusting physiologically, socially, emotionally and psychologically to motherhood. The woman's mood appears to be a barometer, reflecting the baby's needs of feeding, sleeping and crying patterns. The major psychological changes are therefore emotional. New mothers tend to be anxious, oversensitive and easily upset. During this period, exhaustion is a major factor to women's emotional state (Bick et al 2009). This may contribute to alterations in thinking and behaviour as the mother adjusts to the inevitable changes, demands and disruptions to daily life and routine that a new baby brings. One of the most important factors in the woman's regaining a sense of equilibrium over her activities of daily living is her ability to sleep throughout the night. A woman's sexual urges, emotional stability and intellectual acuity may take months, if not longer, to return and for the woman to feel whole again (Raynor 2006).

In the postpartum period, Bryan (2003) reports on the long-term psychosocial impact of multiple births on marital relationship, parental stress and family dynamics. The 24/7 demands of round the clock care for not one but two, three or more babies is utterly exhausting and draining, emotionally and financially. This is bound to affect parents' mood. Add to this mix a woman who is not just older, but who had an operative mode of birth with associated complications. The midwife should consider how her recovery is likely to be affected and her immediate psychological needs in the early days postpartum. Less well understood from the research evidence is whether the interactions between these factors and multiple pregnancy, conspire in some way to contribute to serious mental illness (see Chapter 4). Nonetheless, Cook et al (1998) suggest that in mothers of twins and higher multiples who conceive via IVF, parental stress might be exacerbated if concurrent life stressors co-exist alongside a difficult pregnancy. Increased psychological morbidity is also attributed to these parents' increased expectations of themselves. There is also a higher likelihood for older mothers, and women with twins or higher order multiples to experience a feeling of social isolation. It is essential that the midwife provides practical and emotional support to promote parental self-efficacy and convey to parents that it usually takes time to adapt to the demands of parenthood. Each person adapts at their own individual pace.

Difficult births

Women with multiple gestation and those over 40 years old are more likely to have complications and therefore intensive surveillance during their pregnancy and a cascade of medical interventions. Of course there are some who sail through pregnancy without any problems, and there is always the risk of unnecessary interventions (Huang et al 2008, Hoffman et al 2007). Interventions such as caesarean sections (LSCS) and instrumental vaginal births have a higher association with maternal grief, dissatisfaction and anxiety than a spontaneous vaginal birth. Moreover, LSCS is known to make women psychologically vulnerable, as it induces depression (Fisher et al 1997) and renders women dependent on midwives and loved ones, at least in the initial recovery stages. These women not only lose control over caring for themselves, they need help in caring for their babies. This can affect their sense of self-efficacy, self-esteem and self-confidence. The initiation of breastfeeding can also be difficult, which can compound their feelings of helplessness. All these problems will be magnified in the case of multiple births. A non-judgemental, flexible, supportive and encouraging approach by the midwife is therefore needed. Informing women and their partners antenatally of local support groups such as the Twins and Multiple Births Association (TAMBA) provides hope and real choice.

When a baby dies

A pregnancy loss is a profound experience. A miscarriage, an intrauterine fetal death (IUFD) or a neonatal death (NND) seem a cruel irony, which is always distressing for women, their loved ones and midwives. This unfathomable twist of fate seems even more incomprehensible in the presence of poor obstetric history, previous loss, IVF and loss of a twin, whether spontaneous or selected fetal reduction (**fetocide**) to enhance the chances of a live birth.

Grief can be a complex response to loss when it coincides with pregnancy/birth. When a baby dies the pain of such a loss might lead to delayed or disturbed grief responses. Parents can experience conflicting emotions if they lose a baby from a multiple gestation. On one hand they want to grieve the life that could have been but at the same time they want to rejoice the fact they have a live baby/babies. It is important that the midwife recognises this alongside cultural taboos and influences. She should help parents through the stages of their grief, respect religious beliefs, cultural practice and traditions, recognise her limitations in helping and mobilise assistance from other agencies to support the couple. The midwife has ready access to specialist help from others within the multi-agency and interprofessional teams.

Women who conceive via IVF are known to be more vulnerable to psychological morbidity such as anxiety and depression, and tend to experience a tentative pregnancy as they are more fearful of a pregnancy loss. Midwives need to be available to these women, listening and attending sensitively to their needs. They also need to be conversant with the various grief reactions

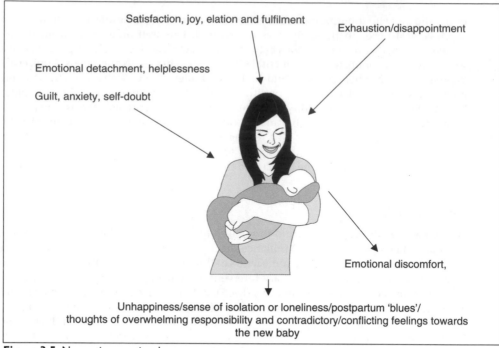

Figure 3.5 Normative emotional responses postpartum

and the psychological implications of multiple gestation and, not least, being an older mother. An understanding of the stresses and strains of assisted reproduction and the toll it takes on couples is also necessary. It should also be noted that marked stress and anxiety during the antenatal period often predicts depressive illness postpartum (Evans et al 2001). The features of postpartum mental illness are discussed in Chapter 4. Figure 3.5 summarises the normative emotional responses that women may experience postpartum.

Family–nurse partnership (FNP)

FNP is a promising area of development that through research has undergone rigorous examination regarding its efficacy (Olds 2006). It is a government initiative where nurses (midwives in some areas) provide intensive home visiting for first-time parents who are young and have known vulnerability factors. The role of FNPs in providing psychosocial support and the benefits of this intervention are explored in greater depth in Chapter 8.

Conclusion

Although it is useful to recognise that motherhood and indeed fatherhood are not biologically determined or socially ascribed, culture, socio-economic means and politics define parenthood. What it means to be a parent, the behaviours and attitudes that define a woman and a man as a 'good' parent or 'bad' parent, will shape their identity, sense of self, relationship with others, the very core of their being and the way in which they are judged by society. Ideals of 'perfection' regarding the female body and its representations can be a distraction for women. Pregnancy, labour, birth and puerperium are times when a woman's profound power and belief in herself further defines her sexuality. These fragile periods are further compounded by biophysical changes, social upheavals and adjustment that a new baby brings. Midwives must be sensitive when communicating and caring for women during these transitional phases. They should be mindful that the transition to parenthood is a particularly charged time emotionally, and that the social context in which children are born will influence the emotional responses of both the mother and father. Having children heaps an immense degree of physical, emotional and social strain on women and their partners that can result in a marked shift in individual life changes, likely to manifest as life events or chronic stressors.

Summary of key points

- Emotions during pregnancy, labour and postpartum are varied, common and contradictory.

- The social construction of motherhood/father is based on a flawed ideology or assumptions and myths.

- The myths of motherhood are presented as:

  - natural
  - instinctive
  - intuitive

- Fatherhood like motherhood is a historical and cultural construct.

- Family life and daily routines are disrupted by the arrival of a new baby.

- Vulnerability factors such as domestic abuse, social adversity associated with lack of social support and poverty, multiple gestations, IVF pregnancies and death of a baby can affect family dynamics and parent–baby relationship.

- The media promotes a romanticised ideology to which all mothers/fathers are supposed to aspire.

- Motherhood and fatherhood are not biologically determined or socially ascribed but are roles defined by culture, socio-economic means and politics.

- Grief is a complex reaction to loss when it coincides with pregnancy/birth.

- What it means to be a mother/father, the behaviours and attitudes that define a woman/ man as a 'good' parent or 'bad' parent will shape their:

  - identity
  - sense of self
  - relationship with others.

References

Barnes, L.D. and Balber, L.G. (2007) *The Journey to Parenthood: myths, reality and what really matters*. Oxford: Radcliffe.

Bewley, S., Ledger, W. and Nikolaou, D. (eds) (2009) *Reproductive Ageing*. London: RCOG.

Bick, D., MacArthur, C., Knowles, H. and Winter, H. (2009) *Postnatal Care: evidence and guidelines for management*, 2nd edn. Edinburgh: Churchill Livingstone.

Boscaglia, N., Skouteris, H. and Wertheim, E.H. (2003) Changes in body image satisfaction during pregnancy: a comparison of high exercising and low exercising women. *Australian and New Zealand Journal of Obstetrics and Gynaecology*, 43(1): 41–5.

Bryan, E. (2003) The impact of multiple preterm births on the family. *British Journal of Obstetrics and Gynaecology*, 110(supplement 20): S24–S28.

Callister, L.C. (1996) Cultural perceptions of childbirth. A cross cultural comparison of childbearing women. *Journal of Holistic Nursing*, 14(1): 66–78.DOI: 10.1177/089801019601400105.

Catch 22 (2009) *Growing up with Dad*. www.catch22.org.uk, accessed 23 March 2009.

Choi, P., Henshaw, C., Baker, S. and Tree, J. (2005) Supermum, superwife, super everything: performing femininity in the transition to motherhood. *Journal of Reproduction and Infant Psychology*, 23(2): 167–80.

Cook, R., Bradley, S. and Colombo, S. (1998) A preliminary study of parental stress and child behaviour in families with twins conceived by in-vitro fertilization. *Human Reproduction*, 13: 3244–6.

Department of Health (2008a) *Getting it Right for Pregnant Teenagers and Young Fathers: a practical guide for midwives, doctors, maternity support workers and receptionists*. London: DH. www.dh.gov.uk, accessed 14 March 2009.

Department of Health (2008b) *Teenage Parents: Who Cares – a guide to commissioning and delivery of maternity services for young parents*. London: Department for Children, Schools and Families, DH, Royal College of Midwives. www.rcm.org.uk, accessed 14 March 2009.

Department of Health (2007a) *Making it Better: for Mother and Baby*. London: DH.

Department of Health (2007b) *Maternity Matters*. London: DH. www.dh.gov.uk, accessed 14 March 2009.

Department of Health (2005) *Responding to Domestic Abuse: a handbook for health professionals*. London: DH. www.dh.gov.uk, accessed 14 March 2009.

Department of Health (2004) *National Service Framework for Children, Young People and Maternity Services*. London: DH. www.dh.gov.uk, accessed 14 March 2009.

Evans, J., Heron, J., Francomb, H., One, S. and Gelding, J. (2001) Cohort study of depressed mood during pregnancy and after childbirth. *British Medical Journal*, 323: 257–60.

Fatherhood Institute (2008) *The Dad Deficit*. www.fatherhoodinstitute.org.uk, accessed 15 March 2009.

Fisher, I.E., Asbury, J. and Smith, A. (1997) Adverse psychological impact of obstetric interventions: a prospective study. *Australian and New Zealand Journal of Psychiatry*, 31: 728–38.

Foresight (2007) *Tackling Obesities – Future Choices Project*. www.foresight.gov.uk, accessed 15 March 2004.

Gilbert, DOT. (2006) *Stumbling on Happiness*. London: Harper.

Grabe, S., Ward, S., Hyde, L.M. and Shipley, J. (2008) The role of media in body image concerns among women: a meta analysis of experimental and correlation studies. *Psychological Bulletin*, 134(3): 460–76.

Grabowska, C. (2009) Unhappiness after childbirth. In: C. Squire (ed.) *The Social Context of Birth*, 2nd edn. Oxford: Radcliffe Press, pp 236–50.

Gross, H. and Pattison, H. (2007) *Sanctioning Pregnancy: a psychological perspective on the paradoxes and culture of research*. London: Routledge.

Hoffman, MAC., Jeffers, S., Carter, J., Dudley, L., Cotter, A. and Gonzalez-Quintero, V.S. (2007) Pregnancy at or beyond age 40 years is associated with an increased risk of fetal death and other adverse outcomes. *American Journal of Obstetrics and Gynaecology*, 196(5): e11–e13.

Home Office (2008) *National Domestic Violence Delivery Plan. Annual progress report 2007/2008*. www.home office.gov.uk, accessed 30 March 2009.

Huang, L., Sauve, R., Birkett, N., Fergusson, D. and van Walraven, C. (2008) Maternal age and risk of stillbirth: a systematic review. *Canadian Medical Association Journal*, 178(2): 165–72.

International Confederation of Midwives (2005) *Definition of the Midwife*. The Hague: ICM.

Jordan, B. (1980) *Birth in Four Cultures: a crosscultural investigation of childbirth in Yucatan, Holland, Sweden and the United States*, 2nd edn. St Albans: Eden Press.

Lewis, G. (ed.) (2007) *Saving Mothers' Lives: reviewing maternal deaths to make motherhood safer 2003–2005*. The seventh report on Confidential Enquiries into Maternal Deaths in the United Kingdom. London: CEMACH.

Lewis, G. and Drife, J. (eds) (2004) *Why Mothers Die 2000–2002*. The sixth report of the Confidential Enquiries into Maternal Deaths in the United Kingdom. London: CEMACH.

Maio, G.R., Haddock, G.G. and Jarman, H.L. (2006) Social psychological factors in tackling obesity. *Obesity Reviews*, 8(Suppl.1): 123–5.

National Institute for Health and Clinical Excellence (2007) *Intrapartum Care: care of healthy women and their babies during childbirth*. CG55. London: NICE.

National Institute for Health and Clinical Excellence (2006) *Routine postnatal care of women and their babies*. CG37. London: NICE.

Nicholson, P. (1997) *Motherhood and Women's Lives*, 2nd edn. London: Macmillan.

Nursing and Midwifery Council (2004) *Midwives Rules and Standards*. London: NMC.

Oakley, A., Hickey, D., Rajan, L. and Rigby, A. (1996) Social support in pregnancy – does it have long term effects? *Journal of Reproduction and Infant Psychology*, 14: 7–22.

Office for National Statistics (2008) *Statistical Bulletin for Births and Deaths in England and Wales*. London: ONS.

Olds, D.L. (2006) The nurse-family partnership: an evidence-based preventive intervention. *Infant Mental Health Journal*, 27(1): 5–25.

O'Reilly, A. (2008) *Feminist Mothering*. Albany: Suny Press.

O'Reilly, A. (2004) *Mother Outlaws: theory and practices of empowered mothering*. Toronto: Women's Press.

Plantin, L. (2007a) Involving men in pregnancy and childbirth. In: World Health Organization 'Is it all about sex? Entrenous' *European Magazine for Sexual and Reproductive Health*, 66: 10–11. www.euro.who.int/entrenous/20020905_1, accessed 20 March 2009.

Plantin, L. (2007b) *Fatherhood and Health Outcomes – the case of Europe*. Copenhagen: WHO. www.euro.who.int, accessed 20 March 2009.

Povey, D. (ed.) (2008) *Homicides, Firearm Offences and Intimate Violence 2006/2007* (supplementary volume 2 to crime in England and Wales 2006/2007) Home Office Statistical Bulletin. www.homeoffice.gov.uk, accessed 22 March 2009.

Powdhavee, N. (2009) Think having children will make you happy? *The Psychologist*, 22(4): 308–10. www.thepsychologist.org.uk, accessed 8 April 2009.

Raynor, M. (2006) Social and psychological context of childbearing. *Women's Health Medicine*, 3(2): 64–7.

Redshaw, M., Rowe, R., Hockley, C. and Brocklehurst, P. (2007) *Recorded Delivery: a national survey of women's experience of maternity care 2006*. Oxford: National Perinatal Epidemiology Unit.

Schwartz, M. and Brownell, K.D. (2004) Obesity and body image. *Journal of Body Image*, 1(1): 43–56.

Silva, E.B. (1996) *Good Enough Mothering? Feminist perspectives on lone motherhood*. London: Routledge.

Skouters, H., Carr, H., Wertheim, E.H., Paxton, S.J. and Duncombe, D. (2005) A prospective study of factors that lead to body dissatisfaction during pregnancy. *Journal of Body Image*, 2(4): 347–61.

Teixeira, J.M.A., Fisk, N.M. and Glover, V. (1999) Association between anxiety in pregnancy and increased uterine artery resistance index: cohort based study. *British Medical Journal* 318: 153–7.

Van den Bergh, B.R., Mulder, E.J., Mennes, M. and Glover, V. (2005) Antenatal maternal anxiety and stress and the neurobehavioural development of the fetus and child: links and possible mechanisms: A review. *Neuroscience Biobehaviour Review*, 29(2): 237–58.

Winson, N. (2009) Transition to motherhood. In: C. Squire (ed.) *The Social Context of Birth*. Oxford: Radcliffe, pp 145–60.

Woolett, A. and Parr, M. (1997) Psychological tasks for women and men in the postpartum. *Journal of Reproductive and Infant Psychology*, 15: 159–83.

World Heath Organization (2009) *Mental health – aspects of women's reproductive health: a global review of the literature*. http://www.who.int, accessed 27 August 2009.

World Health Organization (WHO 2004) *Obesity: preventing and managing the global epidemic*. Report of a WHO consultation. Geneva: WHO. http://www.who.int, accessed 27 April 2009.

Annotated further reading

Bandura, A. (2001) Social cognitive theory: an agentic perspective. *Annual Review in Psychology*, 52: 1–26.

This article explores the importance of being able to exercise control over the nature and quality of one's life/existence.

Paradice, R. (2002) *Psychology for Midwives*. Salisbury: Quay Books.

Useful foundation text.

Rees, M., Karoshi, M. and Keith, L. (2008) *Obesity and Pregnancy*. London: Arnold.

This text address a range of issues around obesity and the childbearing woman including some of the psychological aspects.

Useful websites

www.nice.org.uk
www.who.int
www.rcm.org.uk
www.fatherhoodinstitute.org.uk
www.catch-22.org.uk
www.workingwithmen.org
www.fathersdirect.com
www.harpweb.org.uk
www.hiddenhurt.co.uk

4 Perinatal mental illness

Chapter contents

Introduction

Chapter aims

Clarification of terms

Why maternal mental health matters

Screening for mental illness: prediction and detection

Screening tools

Perinatal psychiatry disorders

Antenatal period – psychiatric disorders in pregnancy

Types of disorder in pregnancy

Serious mental illnesses

Postnatal period: serious psychiatric conditions

Mother–baby relationship

Care/management

Postnatal depressive illnesses

Mother–baby relationship

Care/management

Mild postpartum mood disorders

Mild postnatal depressive illness

Relationship with partner

Role of the midwife: learning lessons from key reports

Managed care networks

Suicide

Medical conditions caused by or mistaken for psychiatric disorder

Sharing best practice

Conclusion

Summary of key points

References

Annotated further reading

Useful websites

Introduction

Perinatal mental illness (PMI) places emphasis on the importance of psychiatric disorder in pregnancy and postpartum. It stems from perinatal psychiatry, a specialist branch of psychiatry dedicated to research, care and treatment of mothers with pre-existing (i.e. preconception) psychiatric illness as well as those arising during pregnancy and **puerperium**. PMI is both a nationally and internationally accepted term; it relates to the effects of mental illness and the implications of treatment on the fetus, breastfeeding and neonatal/child development (Royal College of Psychiatrists (RCPsych) 2000a). This revised terminology highlights the range of mental illness that can affect women during the childbearing years. This means the ubiquitous and erroneous label 'postnatal depression' (PND) is now an outmoded nomenclature, which 'reinforces the view that depression following childbirth is somehow different from depression at other times' (National Institute for Health and Clinical Excellence (NICE) 2007: 38). The chapter will explore the range of psychiatric disorders that midwives need to be conversant with in order to identify those women at risk of serious mental illness (SMI).

Chapter aims

- To discuss the importance of PMI in the maternity context and why maternal mental health matters

- To describe the different types of perinatal psychiatric disorders and their management

- To highlight the implications of PMI on the dynamics of mother/baby relationship

- To examine the role of the midwife in risk assessment/identification

- To highlight lessons to be learnt for midwifery practice from key reports such as the Confidential Enquiries into Maternal and Child Health (CEMACH)

Clarification of terms

Standard terminology is useful both nationally and internationally to prevent misdiagnosis and inappropriate treatment. This will assist the midwife in the identification of conditions that can be easily dealt with in the community setting and those requiring referral and more urgent specialist attention. Like 'PND' use of the term 'mental health problem' is also inappropriate and problematic (Oates and Raynor 2009). Its use in popular culture relates to all types of emotional difficulties from transient and temporary states of distress, which in the maternity context is often understandable, to severe and uncommon mental illness. Its employment over the years has rendered the term non-specific as many extend its use to difficulties coping with the stresses and strains of life, learning difficulties and problems related to substance misuse. The term is too broad, proving of no value to the midwife, failing to discriminate between severity and need. The midwife needs to risk assess and in her decision-making, establish a clear distinction between SMI and milder forms of mental illness. For the purpose of this chapter the revised terminology PMI has been employed instead of 'PND' – a 'cache pot' that fails to recognise that one size does not fit all (Oates 2007).

Why maternal mental health matters

There is a steep rise in the prevalence of psychotic illness, and to a lesser extent, mild to moderate illness associated with having children. Pregnancy is not protective against a **recurrence** or **relapse** of a previous psychiatric disorder particularly if the medication for these disorders is stopped when pregnancy is diagnosed. Childbirth increases the risk of recurrence for women with pre-existing PMI, and for those with SMI, pregnancy and childbirth pose an even greater risk of relapse, which will affect the woman's ability to care for her baby (Oates 2006). Consecutive CEMACH reports emphasise the importance for midwives to make sensitive enquiry about women's current and previous mental health at early pregnancy assessment (Lewis 2007, Lewis and Drife 2001, 2004). The presence of a serious psychiatric disorder during pregnancy and postpartum is a real threat to women's lives and a challenge to the maternity and perinatal mental health service. Policy and service development must therefore address the full range of mental disorders that can occur antenatally and postnatally.

Mental illness affects life chances and is of major public health concern (Department of Health (DH) 2003a). For a number of years it has remained a leading cause of maternal morbidity and mortality in the United Kingdom (UK) (Oates 2001, 2004, 2007). Mental illness during pregnancy and postpartum has huge ramifications not only for the health and wellbeing of the mother but also that of the developing fetus, neonate and family relationships. Infants and children are particularly vulnerable as impaired mental functioning of the mother disrupts not only mother–baby dynamic relationship and interactions but can undermine the social, emotional, cognitive and behavioural development of the infant (Cooper and Murray 1997a). Mental health and wellbeing should, therefore, be core business of the maternity service as it is as important as physical health. In its report on perinatal mental health services the Royal College of Psychiatrists (2000a) justifies the importance of perinatal mental health, as summarised in Box 4.1.

Box 4.1 Why maternal mental health matters (RCPsych 2000a)

- Pregnancy and childbirth provides an excellent and unparalleled opportunity for prevention of a major illness as women are in repeated contact with midwives and other health care professionals.
- The epidemiology of perinatal mental illness in the postnatal period or puerperium is well established. This allows plenty of scope for effective planning of resources.
- The clinical presentation of perinatal psychiatric disorders especially postpartum is well established.
- Factors that increase the risk of non-psychotic postpartum illness can be identified.
- There are adverse consequences for mother and baby if there is a failure to have a proactive management plan to deal with a known perinatal mental illness.
- The risk of **relapse** or **recurrence** of postpartum mental illness is known.
- Effective treatment can be implemented.

Screening for mental illness – prediction and detection

Midwives have an important public health remit (DH 2001). They work across a wide spectrum and are able to engage in a coordinated way with other disciplines to make a substantial contribution to the wider public health agenda. A plethora of social policies have identified the need to improve the quality of services through increased choice and access to midwives, especially those women who are vulnerable and disadvantaged (DH 2003a, 2003b, 2004, 2007a, 2007b). Consequently, midwives are now the first point of contact for many pregnant women (DH 2007a). Not only do midwives need a good working knowledge and essential skills training in order to recognise the normative adjustment reactions involved in the transition to motherhood (Chapter 3), they also need to be skilled at identifying early those women at risk of developing a serious or major psychiatric disorder.

The importance of antenatal screening to detect a history of previous mental illness, its severity, the form of care the woman received in order to establish how the illness was managed and the risk of recurrence has been highlighted (NICE 2006, 2007, 2008, Lewis 2007, DH 2004, Lewis and Drife 2001, 2004, Scottish Intercollegiate Guidelines Network Group [SIGN] 2002). NICE (2007) *Antenatal and Postnatal Mental Health* guideline states that at a woman's initial contact with services in both the antenatal and postnatal periods, healthcare professionals (including midwives, obstetricians, health visitors and general practitioners) should ask specific questions about:

- past or present SMI (i.e. schizophrenia, bipolar disorder, psychosis in the postnatal period and unipolar severe depression)
- previous treatment by a psychiatrist/specialist mental health team including inpatient care
- a family history of serious PMI.

Screening tools

The Whooley questions

To assess maternal emotional wellbeing, NICE (2007) recommends use of the 'Whooley' questions (Figure 4.1). This is based on a two-question case-finding instrument to detect depression, which emerged from a scientific study conducted by Whooley et al (1997). The researchers concluded that using the two questions has the advantage of being less time consuming when compared to other case-finding instruments with similar test characteristics that asks about depressed mood and **anhedonia**. They also suggested that these two brief focused questions that address mood and interest are as likely to be as effective as more elaborate methods for identifying depression, and are more compatible with routine use in many primary and secondary care settings. NICE (2007) added a third question as outlined in Figure 4.1.

Edinburgh postnatal depression scale (EPDS)

The EPDS is a simple 10-item questionnaire intended to be capable of completion in 5 minutes. The aim of this risk assessment tool is to assist health visitors to detect mothers with postnatal depressive illness. Cox et al (1987) developed the scale for research purposes for use postpartum, and referred to published work demonstrating 10–15% of mothers experience a marked depressive illness in the months following childbirth. At least half of these mothers have not recovered by the end of the postpartum year, and the children of such depressed mothers may show behavioural disturbances at 3 years or cognitive defects at 4 years. The second or third month postpartum is the best time to administer the questionnaire. Scores for each item range from 0 to 3 according to severity. Cox et al (1987) suggested a threshold of 12/13 being a predictive risk, and women scoring above this are most likely to be suffering from a depressive illness. Although the **validity** of the EPDS has been tested on a large community sample (Murray and Caruthers 1990) it should be used with caution. This is a predictive rather than diagnostic test, and women's psychological wellbeing will require further assessment to confirm whether or not they are clinically depressed (Cox and Holden 1994). An 11/12 cut off threshold has been highlighted as having a **specificity** of 92.5%, a predictive value of 35.1% and a **sensitivity** of 88% (Cooper and Murray 1997b). A threshold of 10 is used by specialist community nurses/health visitors. However, concerns have been raised about the misuse and limitations that the EPDS affords in primary care (Leverton and Elliot 2000, Elliot 1994). Cantwell (2003) asserts that a good screening test should reflect both reliability and validity. The National Screening Committee (2001) calls for more work in relation to use of the EPDS, concluding that it is important to determine its validity in routine primary care, and expressing concerns about its widespread implementation as a screening tool for 'PND' throughout the UK. It is worth remembering a score on a screening tool is not the same as a clinical diagnosis (Oates and Raynor 2009).

The following questions must take into account the woman's socio-cultural background:

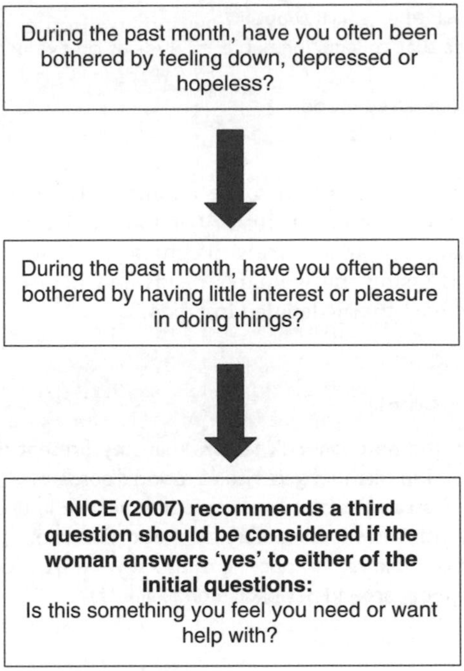

During the past month, have you often been bothered by feeling down, depressed or hopeless?

⬇

During the past month, have you often been bothered by having little interest or pleasure in doing things?

⬇

NICE (2007) recommends a third question should be considered if the woman answers 'yes' to either of the initial questions:
Is this something you feel you need or want help with?

Figure 4.1 The 'Whooley' Questions (NICE 2007)

Risk factors

Risk factors are best construed as adverse or vulnerability factors, hazards, variables or indeed characteristics that feature in an individual's life and put them at risk of illness. Risk factors are useful as a correlation but are not necessarily causal; meaning the presence of a risk factor might not result in illness though a cluster of these adverse factors increases the individual's vulnerability. Although numerous studies such as Beck (2001), O'Hara and Swain (1996), Murray et al (1995) and Cox et al (1993) identified various risk factors associated with PMI (Box 4.2), it appears that different risk factors have different effects. This is dictated by timing or when they manifest during pregnancy and postpartum. Thus the evidence to support the role of some risk factors as independent variables is weak.

Box 4.2 Potential risk factors for mood disorders during the perinatal period (Beck 2001, Cooper and Murray 1997b, O'Hara and Swain 1996, Murray et al 1995):

- Previous history of a depressive illness, especially during the perinatal period;
- Psychosocial adversity that is persistent or enduring (e.g. assisted reproduction techniques such as IVF pregnancy, caring for a sick relative, poverty and unemployment);

- Unwanted pregnancy; as cited in the CEMACH report (Lewis 2007) the risk is manifold where termination is considered and rejected.
- Lack of a confidante or social support.
- Personality type that reflects inflexible, rigid ideals or overly conscientiousness always striving for perfection.
- Presence of a depressed mood.

Midwives should be conversant with the potential risk factors that may be associated with antecedent factors such as previous history of a mood disorder, especially during the perinatal period. Factors that may arise during pregnancy, labour and postpartum should also be considered when assessing the woman's needs and planning care. The reader is invited to complete the reflective activity detailed in Box 4.3.

Box 4.3 Reflective activity

1. Make a list of the potential risk factors that may present during pregnancy, labour and the postpartum period that may give risk to mood disorders.
2. Identify helpful strategies that may assist the midwife in providing effective care for women who present with known risk factors for mood disorders.
3. Make a list of the voluntary support groups known to you locally that the woman could enlist to provide support around perinatal mental illness.

Perinatal psychiatry disorders

Emotional difficulties during pregnancy and puerperium represent a wide variation between individual women. They range from minor transient disturbance with rapid unaided adjustment through common mental disorders to severe or SMI such as **puerperal psychosis** – an acute and distressing psychiatric emergency. Although the range and types of mental illness are very varied, these illnesses form part of a continuum. All psychiatric disorders can present in pregnancy and postpartum as women with the whole range of psychiatric disorders become pregnant and have children (NICE 2007). Although the early postnatal period can be a time of great joy and personal fulfilment for many mothers, pregnancy, childbirth and the demands of 24-hour care generated by a dependent baby may precipitate problems. It may lead a woman to seek help for her longstanding difficulties at this time (Oates 2006). The evidence that untreated mental disorder in pregnancy may be associated with poorer long-term outcomes for children beyond the immediate postnatal period is of concern. Midwives should understand the negative consequences of impaired maternal–baby interactions and negative perceptions of infant behaviour as notable vulnerability factors (Cooper and Murray 1997a, Murray and Cooper 2003).

Prevalence

The **prevalence** of psychiatric disorders relates to the total number of individuals ill at any given time, and includes old and new illnesses. As reported by the Office of National Statistics (ONS 2002) psychiatric disorders are very common in the general population with a prevalence of over 20%. Studies have identified that the majority of psychiatric disorders in society are mild to moderate conditions, particularly general anxiety and depression (Cox et al 1993,

O'Hara and Swain 1996). Mild to moderate depressive illness and anxiety disorders are at least twice as common in women than in men, and are particularly common in young women with children under the age of 5 (Oates 2006). Clearly, having children puts a woman at greater risk of developing a mental illness than at other times in her life. Oates (1996) observed that the chances of women developing a form of SMI following childbirth, and being admitted to hospital, is significantly increased when compared with men and women in the general population. Brown et al (2005) state that the majority of mood disorders stem from stress factors associated with social inequality such as poverty and isolation. All pregnancies carry risks but these risks increase where the woman is mentally ill.

Incidence

Incidence (new onset) relates to the number of individuals who become ill who have been previously well. In pregnancy the most common psychiatric disorders encountered are mild depression, anxiety or mixed anxiety and depression states (Oates 2006). Estimate of the incidence of mild affective states such as depression and anxiety in pregnancy is identified as being approximately 10–15% (Kumar and Robson 1984). It is vital that the midwife recognises that some women may experience a recurrence of these conditions whilst pregnant. This may be triggered by social adversity or other vulnerability factors such as previous pregnancy loss, having no supportive partner, socio-economic hardship and previous fertility problems. In contrast to the puerperium, there is no evidence that the incidence of SMI is elevated during pregnancy. However, while the incidence of SMI appears to be lower in pregnancy than at other times (Kendell et al 1987) pregnancy does not appear protective of risk of a recurrence or relapse of a pre-existing illness.

More than 10% of women following birth will experience a new episode of depressive illness. Oates (2006) states that in the case of depressive illness all severities are represented in women who have previously been well. O'Hara and Swain (1996) reflect that approximately 3% of women will experience moderate to severe depression and Kendell et al (1987) identify 0.2% will suffer from puerperal psychosis, the rarest of postpartum mental disorders (Robertson et al 2005).

Table 4.1 identifies the conventional categories in which psychiatric disorders are placed.

Table 4.1 Types or categories of psychiatric disorders (Oates and Raynor 2009)

1. Serious mental illnesses

Previously known as psychotic disorders include:

- schizophrenia
- bipolar illness
- severe (unipolar) depressive illness
- other psychotic conditions.

2. Mild to moderate psychiatric disorders

Previously referred to in the psychiatric literature as 'neurotic disorders' include:

- panic disorder
- non-psychotic mild to moderate depressive illness
- mixed anxiety and depression
- anxiety disorders including:
  - phobic anxiety states
  - obsessive compulsive disorder (OCD)
  - post-traumatic stress disorder (PTSD).

Table 4.1—*continued*

3. Adjustment reactions

This category encompasses distressing reactions to life events or life crises e.g. marital strife/separation, bereavement and other social adversity.

4. Substance misuse

Includes those individuals who misuse or who are dependent upon substances such as alcohol and other drugs of dependency including both prescription and legal/illegal drugs.

5. Personality disorders

A term loosely used in the general population but which should only be used to describe those individuals who have enduring and severe problems throughout their adult life in dealing with the stresses and strains of normal life. This includes:

- difficulty in controlling their behaviour
- difficulty in maintaining satisfactory relationships
- acting irresponsibly and failing to foresee the consequences of their own actions
- persistently causing distress to themselves and other people.

6. Learning disability

A term used to describe individuals who portray evidence of intellectual and cognitive impairment, developmental delay and consequent learning disabilities throughout their life time. Learning disability is usually graded as:

- – mild
- – moderate
- – severe.

Antenatal period – psychiatric disorders in pregnancy

Psychiatric disorders do not discriminate between the pregnant/non-pregnant states; all the psychiatric disorders detailed in Table 4.1 do complicate pregnancy and the puerperium. During pregnancy some women will be taking antidepressants, mood stabilisers or other psychotropic medication used to treat psychiatric disorders. Only a small proportion of women will have a past history of a SMI and will currently be suffering from such an illness. Pregnancy does not appear to be protective against a recurrence or relapse of a previous psychiatric disorder. Midwives must therefore encourage women who are on medication not to stop taking them. If the midwife or woman is unsure whether such medications are contraindicated during pregnancy, guidance must be sought from either the general practitioner or psychiatrist treating the woman. Midwives also need to know that women with a past history of SMI during the puerperium or at other times are at increased risk of a recurrence of that illness. Oates (2006) identifies this risk as being 1:2 to 1:3.

Types of disorder in pregnancy

Mild to moderate mental illnesses

As previously stated, the majority of psychiatric disorders within the population are mild to moderate conditions, which are mainly:

- general anxiety and depression
- mild depressive illness
- mixed anxiety and depression
- anxiety states.

These conditions usually present in the early trimesters of pregnancy and are less common in the third trimester. The cause is unclear with extensive studies suggesting a range of contributory factors (Dennis 2005). However, what is consistently identified via the evidence from epidemiological research and meta-analyses of predictive studies is the part played by psychosocial risk factors (Beck 2001, Cooper and Murray 1997b, O'Hara and Swain 1996) as previously outlined in Box 4.2. These include life crises such as poor/lack of social support, marital discord, other life stressors and reasons for personal unhappiness that may be precipitated by low maternal self-esteem (Jomeen and Martin 2005).

Care/management

According to Cooper and Murray (1997b) and Oates (2006) the majority of mild to moderate conditions are likely to improve as pregnancy advances, and are managed in primary care as they do not require the attention of specialist psychiatric services. NICE (2007) recommends psychological therapies for the management of such conditions, which seem to respond favourably to these treatments. However, each case must be assessed individually on a case by case basis and the choice of treatment governed by factors such as efficacy, compliance and women's preference (NICE 2007, SIGN 2002). The psychiatrist or GP treating the woman needs to exercise caution before pharmacological interventions are used during pregnancy to ensure safety for the mother and developing fetus. The issue of safety also needs careful consideration to balance risks and benefits if the woman plans to breastfeed.

Prognosis

Antenatally, not only do mild to moderate conditions respond well to psychological treatments, the conditions usually improve over the course of the pregnancy. For those women who are mentally unwell in the latter stages of their pregnancy, their psychiatric condition is likely to continue into the postnatal period (Oates 2006).

Serious mental illnesses

The varied conditions that are categorised as SMI are listed in Table 4.1. They are uncommon in pregnancy because they are less common in the general population. Only 1% of the population is affected by **schizophrenia** and **bipolar illness** (Oates 2006). Bipolar illness affects men and women equally, with the exception of schizophrenia, particularly the more severe chronic forms, which affect more men than women. During pregnancy and postpartum the presence of SMI will require the expertise and attention of specialist perinatal psychiatric service, where pharmacological treatments, comprehensive specialist care including psychological therapy, can be implemented. Each National Health Service (NHS) Trust within the UK must have a defined pathway of care for these women (Lewis 2007, NICE 2007, DH 2004, Lewis and Drife 2004, RCPsych 2000a). A history of SMI during an antenatal 'booking' history is sufficient reason for the midwife to make a referral to the perinatal psychiatric service, as this is the group of women CEMACH (Lewis and Drife 2004, Lewis 2007) and SIGN (2002) highlight being most at risk of suicide.

Incidence

Women are at a lower risk of developing an SMI during pregnancy than at other times in their lives. This is in marked contrast to the elevated risk of suffering from such a condition in the first few months following childbirth (Kendell et al 1987). These conditions albeit rare require urgent and specialist treatment via the perinatal mental health service. An acute psychosis in pregnancy poses a real risk to the mother and developing fetus, both directly because of the disturbed behaviour and indirectly because of the pharmacological treatments (Oates 2006).

Three broad groups of women are described by Oates (2006) as follows:

Group 1: women who have had a previous episode of bipolar illness or a psychotic episode earlier in their lives. These women are usually stable, not on medication and well enough to not be in contact with psychiatric services. If their last episode of illness was more than two years ago they may not be at an increased risk of a **recurrence** of their condition during pregnancy but face at least a 50% risk of becoming psychotic in the early weeks postpartum. The most important aspect of management is for there to be a proactive management plan for the first few weeks following birth. Early risk identification and referral by the midwife to the perinatal psychiatric team is therefore pivotal.

Group 2: applies to women who have had a previous and/or recent episode of an SMI, who are relatively well and stable but who are medicated to help maintain health and wellbeing. This may be psychotropic (antipsychotic) medication or in the case of bipolar illness, a mood stabiliser e.g. lithium carbonate or carbamepazine (also used as an anticonvulsant). These women are at risk of a relapse of their condition during pregnancy, which is particularly high if they stop their medication at the diagnosis of pregnancy. As some of these medications may have an adverse effect on the development of the fetus and yet an acute relapse of the illness also is hazardous, it is important that these women have access to expert advice. A perinatal psychiatrist is best placed to provide care and guidance on the risks and benefits of continuing the treatment or changing it as early as possible antenatally.

Group 3: relates to the broad group of women who are chronically mentally ill with complex social needs, persisting symptoms and on medication. The midwife should be aware that these women will usually be in contact with psychiatric services. A joined-up approach to interprofessional working between psychiatric, midwifery and obstetric care is necessary to ensure good integration and no omission in care of these women. Effective multidisciplinary working and partnership is also needed between the named midwife, GP, obstetrician, psychiatrist, health visitor and social services.

Need for proactive management plan

Relevant CEMACH reports (Lewis and Drife 2004, Lewis 2007) and NICE (2007) guidelines have made clear that for optimum care all women who have a current or previous history of SMI should have advice and counselling before planning a pregnancy. Such pre-pregnancy counselling should include discussion around:

- risk to their mental health of becoming pregnant
- the demands of parenthood and the emotional changes that take place during this time
- the risks to the developing fetus of continuing with their usual medication and perhaps the need to review or change it to avoid teratogenesis.

Such an optimistic plan and proactive approach is difficult to materialise because in the general population a vast number of pregnancies are unplanned at the point of conception. Midwives making sensitive enquiry at first contact with the woman about her previous and current psychiatric history are likely to ensure that the psychiatric services are alerted early about the pregnancy. This is critical in order to prevent relapses of the psychiatric illness during pregnancy and recurrences postpartum.

Postnatal period: serious psychiatric conditions

Puerperal psychosis

Puerperal psychosis is the least common of postpartum conditions and is an acute psychiatric emergency. The condition has been recognised and described since antiquity. It is also regarded as the most florid, severe and dramatic form of postpartum affective disorder (Kendell et al 1987).

Incidence

It leads to 2 per 1000 women being admitted to a psychiatric hospital following childbirth, mostly in the first few weeks postpartum. Although a relatively rare condition, it is a major reason for psychotic illness following childbirth (Kendell et al 1987). It is also remarkably constant across nations and cultures (Robertson et al 2005).

Risk factors

The majority of women who are affected by this condition will have been previously well, without obvious risk factors and the illness comes as a shock to them and their family. Some women will have a recurrence of the illness having suffered from a similar episode after the birth of a previous child. Others may have suffered from a non-postpartum bipolar affective disorder from which they have long recovered (see Case scenario 4.1) or they may have a family history of bipolar illness. Robertson et al (2005) provide evidence that a family history of bipolar disorder is a simple clinical variable that may be of prognostic value; marked psychosocial adversity might also be present.

Case scenario 4.1 History of bipolar illness

Yasmin is a 37-year-old IT consultant who is pregnant with her first child following fertility treatment. She lives with her partner Richard, a property developer. The couple recently purchased a large house and relocated to a new area. They now live over 100 miles away from their friends and respective families. At the antenatal 'booking' Yasmin disclosed to the midwife that she has suffered bipolar illness in the past but has been well for the past 10 years.

Key discussion points

1. What are the main risk factors identified by this scenario?
2. What is the risk of recurrence of bipolar illness postpartum?
3. What actions should the midwife take?
4. Read NICE (2007) antenatal and postnatal mental health guidelines and discuss the care pathway that should be in place to care for Yasmin during pregnancy and postpartum periods.
5. What support should be in place for Richard?

Aetiology

Puerperal psychosis appears to be much less related to stress or psychosocial adversity and more related to biochemical changes. Biological factors (neuroendocrine and genetic) are cited as the most important aetiological factors for this condition (Kendell et al 1987). The strong association between family history of bipolar illness and puerperal psychosis suggests a genetic link (Oates 1996), and justifies asking about a family history of SMI at antenatal booking. It also implies that puerperal psychosis can and does strike without warning affecting women across the social spectrum.

Clinical features

The features of this acute and early onset condition are florid and dramatic (see Figure 4.2), tending to change rapidly and altering from day to day during the acute phase of the illness, with the overwhelming majority of cases presenting in the first two weeks postpartum (Kendell et al 1987). Symptoms rarely arise within 48 hours following birth and most commonly develop suddenly between days 3 and 7, at a time when most women will be experiencing the postnatal 'blues'. Thus it may be challenging to make a differential diagnosis between the earliest phase of a developing psychosis and the 'blues'. Nonetheless, the midwife should bear in mind that

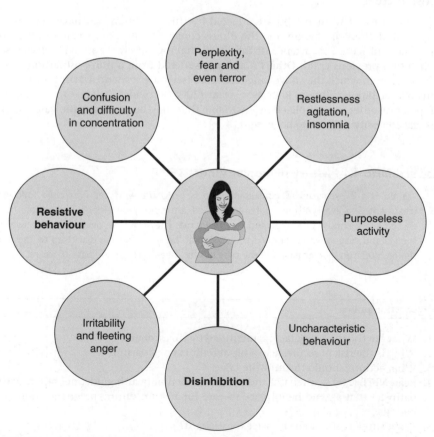

Figure 4.2 Common and early features of puerperal psychosis

while puerperal psychosis steadily deteriorates over the initial 48 hours, the 'blues' tends to resolve spontaneously (Oates 2006).

During the first 2 to 3 days of a developing puerperal psychosis there is a fluctuating rapidly changing, undifferentiated psychotic state. Figure 4.2 identifies some of the more common and earliest features of the condition.

As the woman's condition deteriorates she is likely to be gripped by psychosis (**hallucinations** and **delusions**) and bizarre delusions, e.g. the woman may believe that she is still pregnant or that the baby is not hers. Also it is not unusual for the motives and identity of loved ones and healthcare professionals to be mistaken or misinterpreted in a delusional manner. The woman may have fears for her own and her baby's health and safety, or even about its identity. A state of perplexity and terror is often found. A blend of grandiosity, elation and certain conviction alternating with states of confusion, disorientation, tearfulness, guilt and a sense of foreboding are not uncommon. Suspiciousness and depression may also dominate.

Women affected by puerperal psychosis are among the most profoundly disturbed and distressed found in psychiatric practice (Robertson et al 2005). Most women will present with features suggestive of a depressive psychosis with a significant minority experiencing signs of mania. More commonly they will have a mixture of both – a mixed affective psychosis, pressure of speech and flight of ideas (Oates 2006). Other features often include restlessness, agitation, **resistive behaviour** and the woman seeking senselessly to escape and difficult to reassure. However, the presence and familiarity of loved ones can be a calming influence. Marked deterioration in the woman's mental functioning often leads to a gross impairment in her concentration. She is severely tested to the extent that her ability to care for her baby and attend to her personal hygiene and nutrition is affected. Further, impaired concentration makes her easily distractible and unable to undertake and complete the simplest of tasks.

Mother–baby relationship

An inability to complete and organise day-to-day tasks and routines may also result in unintentional neglect of the baby, which might be misconstrued by well-intentioned healthcare professionals that the baby is at risk of harm from the mother. Some mothers are unaware that the baby is theirs, while others are preoccupied with the baby, reluctant to let it out of their sight and repeatedly checking on its presence and wellbeing. Delusional ideas may frequently involve the baby such as notions around ill health or changed identity (Oates and Raynor 2009). It is rare indeed for women with puerperal psychosis to exact punitive or aggressive behaviour towards their baby (Appleby et al 1994). The risk to the baby lies more from the mother's inability to organise and complete tasks due to her impaired mental state (Oates 2006). These problems are directly attributable to the maternal psychosis and will resolve as the mother recovers. The most important factors in minimising risk are fourfold:

- prompt detection
- appropriate referral
- early intervention
- timely, effective, sensitive but speedy management.

Care/management

Women with puerperal psychosis require urgent admission to hospital. The gold standard of care should involve admission to a specialist perinatal mother and baby unit, where there are perinatal psychiatrists and specialist psychiatric nurses. Although this is the only setting in which the physical needs of the mother who has recently given birth and her baby can be met (Lewis 2007, NICE 2007, SIGN 2002, RCPsych 2000a), nationally there is a shortage of perinatal mother and baby units (RCPsych 2000b). Skilled and empathetic care is vital, as it is usually difficult for the woman and her family to accept symptoms and diagnosis of a psychotic illness. This model of care will ensure a thorough assessment of the mother's ability to care for her baby and will foster the mother–baby relationship in a therapeutic environment. Family therapy can also occur and will serve to provide insight and understanding regarding the behaviour and needs of the distressed and acutely ill mother.

Prognosis

With early recognition and prompt appropriate treatment, the florid and distressing features of puerperal psychosis usually resolve relatively quickly over 2–4 weeks. Initial recovery is often fragile and the risk of a relapse is high in the first few weeks (Oates 2006). Resolution of the psychosis results in women commonly passing through a phase of depression and anxiety. Preoccupation with their past experiences and the implications of these memories for their future mental health and their role as a mother also ensue. Despite the gravity of the illness the prospects for recovery is excellent. The overwhelming majority of women will make good progress and would have completely recovered by 3–6 months postpartum. However, there is at least a 50% risk of a recurrence following the birth of another child, and a strong possibility that some will develop bipolar illness at other times in their lives (Robertson et al 2005). Women need counselling and skilled help during this critical period to help them make sense of what has happened. Information about the risks of a relapse and recurrence of the illness should be provided in a sensitive and non-alarmist way (Cantwell and Smith 2006).

Postnatal depressive illnesses

As stated earlier, more than 10% of all women who have recently given birth will develop a depressive illness. This figure is derived from community studies using the EPDS either as a diagnostic tool or as a screening tool prior to the use of other research tools. NICE (2007) stresses that depression following childbirth has the same subtypes along a spectrum of severity as depression at other times. Depending on their symptomatology, severity and onset, depressive illnesses following childbirth may be graded as mild to moderate or severe, and subtypes may have prominent anxiety and obsessional phenomena (Oates 2006, Cooper and Murray 1995). It can be concluded that a depressive illness following childbirth is relatively common and with the exception of the most severe forms, it is no more common in pregnancy than among women of childbearing years in the general population (O'Hara and Swain 1996). However, due to the maternity context when there are major psychological upheavals and women have to adjust to the demands of their new mothering role, depression at this transitional phase in women's lives is indeed testing.

Severe (unipolar) depressive illness

Major depression may occur in the first month postpartum, at a time when midwives traditionally are withdrawing care, and may last for months (Oates 2006). Cox et al (1993) point to a 7-fold increase in risk in the first 3 months following birth of women developing a severe depressive illness. Affonso et al (2000) and Kumar (1994) found that depression is a major mental health issue for many women from diverse ethnicities and cultures.

Incidence

With its biological features this illness is known to affect at least 3% of all postpartum women. Similar to other mental illnesses that present postpartum the majority of women who suffer from this condition will have been previously well. However, women with a previous history of severe postnatal depressive illness or severe depression at other times or a family history of severe depressive illness, including postpartum, are at increased risk.

Risk factors

As stated previously, Beck (2001), Evans et al (2001), Cooper and Murray (1998, 1997b) and O'Hara and Swain (1996) have all identified several risk factors for postnatal depressive illness, which are associated with depression at other times (Box 4.2). Oates (2006) also added a few others such as ambivalence about the pregnancy, high levels of anxiety during pregnancy and adverse birth experiences. The statistical significant and positive predictive value of these all too common risk factors is unclear. However, the midwife should not discount a clustering of these risk factors but should recognise the importance of being more vigilant when caring for women postnatally. Risk factors that have a higher positive predictive value are deemed more relevant (Oates 2006). These include a family history of severe affective disorder or severe postnatal depressive illness, developing a depressive illness in the last trimester of pregnancy and the loss of the previous infant (including stillbirth). Pregnancies resulting from in vitro fertilisation (IVF) are also considered to be an added risk factor.

Aetiology

The actual cause of the illness is unclear, and although biological factors play an important role in the most severe illnesses, psychosocial factors are more important in the aetiology of this condition than in puerperal psychosis.

The onset of severe depressive illness is early and similar to puerperal psychosis but more insidious in nature as it often starts gradually in the first 2–4 postpartum weeks. At the more severe end of the spectrum the illness is more likely to present early and will be evident by 4–6 weeks postpartum. Nonetheless in the majority of cases the presentation is later, usually between 8 and 12 weeks postpartum, in which case the illness may be missed. Oates and Raynor (2009) provide an explanation that some of the symptoms may be misattributed to the normal transition that the mother has to make as she adjusts to her new baby and mothering role. A further explanation could be attributed to the mother not wanting to be judged as a 'bad' mother and pretending that she is coping in order to conceal her true feelings from others.

Clinical features

Oates (2006) states that the familiar symptoms of severe depressive illness are often modified by the early weeks and demands of motherhood as well as the relative youth of childbearing women affected by the condition; Box 4.4 summarises the main features of severe postpartum depressive illness.

Box 4.4 Main features of severe postpartum depressive illness (Oates 2006)

- Emotional detachment and profound lowering of mood;
- Loss of appetite and weight;
- Impaired concentration and fearfulness;
- Agitation and restlessness;
- Slowing of mental functioning and mother may become indecisive and withdrawn;
- Lethargy and lack of drive;
- 'Somatic syndrome' of broken sleep and early morning wakening with diurnal variation of mood i.e. the woman will feel most depressed and her symptoms will be worst at the start of the day;
- Pervasive **anhedonia** or loss of pleasure that often lead to feelings of guilt, incompetence and unworthiness;
- Some mothers may find it difficult to engage with the daily task of caring for the baby while others might be fiercely protective of the baby;
- Problems with establishing breastfeeding that are quite common in new mothers may become the subject of morbid rumination;
- The mother may misattribute normal infant behaviour to mean that the baby is suffering or does not like her.

Variations: anxiety and obsessive compulsive symptoms

The majority of postpartum onset mental illnesses are affective (mood) disorders. However, symptoms other than those due to a disorder of mood are frequently present. Severe anxiety, panic attacks and obsessional compulsive symptomatology are common following birth. Women with pre-existing anxiety, panic disorder or obsessional compulsive disorder (OCD) will often experience a relapse or recurrence of their symptoms postpartum (Oates and Raynor 2009).

Incidence

It is not known from the literature whether there is an increase in incidence of these conditions following childbirth.

Clinical features

Phobic anxiety, panic disorders and OCD might be a variation on a theme. Oates (2006) notes symptoms can dominate the clinical picture or accompany a depressive illness postpartum. Anxiety might be the prevailing feature leading to feelings of apprehension, palpitations, tension headaches and dizziness. An acute episode of anxiety associated with intense fear of losing control, hyperventilating or over-breathing is called a panic attack. These symptoms can be triggered when the woman is out shopping or travelling on public transport leading to **agoraphobia**. This may result in the woman not wanting to leave her home; hence a habit of avoidance soon sets in. Symptoms experienced by sufferers can be so distressing that they frequently underpin mental health crises and general calls for emergency attention and maternal fears for the baby. Other features are summarised in Box 4.5.

> **Box 4.5 Some additional features of anxiety and obsessive compulsive states**
>
> - Thoughts that are repetitive intrusive, and often deeply repugnant.
> - Ruminative thoughts may involve harm coming to the baby or loved ones.
> - Intrusive thoughts may lead to repetitive doubting and checking.
> - Feelings of self-doubt may dominate where the woman may feel unable to care for the baby – that she is unsafe as a mother and believes that she is capable of harming her offspring.
> - Tumultuous feelings of anxiety and panic attacks may be precipitated by simple acts such as the baby's crying or being difficult to settle.
> - A crying or unsettled baby may result in the woman feeling fearful to embrace the task of childcare whilst alone. Unfortunately such an expression of fear is often misunderstood and can be too often misinterpreted by professionals who may fear that the baby is at risk.
> - Excessive cleanliness and, like the disproportionate anxiety about the baby, there may also be an obsession with personal health and hygiene.

Mother–baby relationship

Some women with symtomatology of severe depressive illness can find that their feelings and mood have a profound effect on the relationship with the baby, especially when marked anxiety and OCD also features. The majority of mothers who experience a severe depressive illness postpartum are usually vigilant in ensuring that their baby is physically well cared for. The fear experienced by these mothers from their intrusive thoughts and negative feelings can be overwhelming, leaving them frightened and subject to experiencing pervasive anhedonia or loss of pleasure when caring for their baby. Understandably many of those affected will have a profound sense of guilt and unworthiness as they doubt their ability to mother their baby. Timely recognition and treatment are necessary for recovery of the mother and normal cognitive, emotional and social development of the child (Cooper and Murray 1997a).

Care/management

Although the treatment for depressive illness postpartum is no different to depression at other times, speedy resolution of severe depressive illness in the maternity context will result from input from a specialist perinatal mental health team. NICE (2007) cites good recovery by the mother with use of appropriate antidepressant therapy combined with psychological treatments such as psychotherapy.

Prognosis

Appropriate treatment will enable a full recovery, but spontaneous resolution will be more protracted without timely treatment, and may take many months for women to recover. Oates (2006) states a third of women can still be ill when their child is one year old. Cooper and Murray (1995) identify that in the case of severe (unipolar) depression, women with a known history face a 1:2 to 1:3 risk of a recurrence of the illness following the birth of subsequent children. Moreover these women are also at increased risk from suffering from a depressive illness at other times in their lives. Robling et al (2000) suggest the long-term prognosis appears more positive postpartum than when the first episode is in non-childbearing women, both in terms of the frequency of further episodes and in their overall functioning.

Mild postpartum mood disorders

This section of the chapter will examine the following areas: constraints of the medical model drawing on a feminist paradigm to inform the discourse, emotional distress associated with traumatic birth events, the postnatal 'blues' and mild depressive illness that may present postpartum.

Constraints of the medical model: a feminist perspective

Pregnancy and childbirth bring episodes of repeated contact between the woman, midwives and other healthcare professionals, providing unprecedented opportunity to explore the woman's feelings, experience and emotions (RCPsych 2000a). Undoubtedly this opportunity should be readily grasped by midwives as it is a time when explanations provided antenatally about the transition to parenthood and the emotions involved can be reinforced through parent education classes (Barlow et al 2002). Equally it is important to recognise normative emotional reactions to change from those of pathological adjustments in order that women's moods are not homogenised and medicalised. Women's moods when viewed within the constraints of the medical model tend to be confining, one-dimensional and rigid in its approach. This perspective Choi et al (2005), Nicholson (1998) plus Barclay and Lloyd (1996) contend, fails to validate and harmonise the depth of women's feelings. As discussed in Chapter 3, a number of feminist researchers contest the social construction of motherhood and the whole ideology of womanhood. Ussher (1992), Phoenix and Woollett (1991) as well as Nicholson (1998) offer an alternative view on women's emotions following childbirth that is commonly labelled as mild depressive illness. They suggest that women's reactions to motherhood are not always a positive experience as many factors may collide and collude in contributing to unhappiness following childbirth (Winson 2009). The suggested 'depressive' symptoms postpartum may be features of maternal adaptation to the mothering role as women grieve for the loss of their former self – their identity, and adjust to the conflicting demands heaped on them by virtue of their position in society. The dangers of labelling, misdiagnosis and misuse of terminology can do inexplicable damage from the viewpoint of a woman's mental health.

Emotional distress associated with traumatic birth events

Understanding the root cause and expression of mental distress associated with pregnancy and childbirth is complex. It is important to recognise the inter-relationship between traumatic life events and women's mental health especially those events that might lead to post traumatic stress disorder (PTSD) (Lyons 1998). There is now a website specifically related to birth trauma: www.birthtraumaassociation.org.uk. Trauma during childbirth mars a woman's experience from what is meant to be one of the happiest days in her life to one of anguish, pain and distress. Effects of intense pain, use of technological interventions, poor communication, insensitive and disrespectful care may prove very distressing and frightening as tellingly depicted within Case scenario 4.2.

Case scenario 4.2 An example of emotional distress

Izumi is keen to have a natural labour and birth utilising hypnobirthing techniques. However, her labour was induced at 43 weeks. She went on to have all the medical interventions that her birth plan reflected that she did not want i.e. electronic fetal monitoring, artificial rupture of the membranes, intravenous infusion, an epidural, being confined to the bed and the birth culminating in an emergency caesarean section. This was further compounded by labour suite being very busy negating the 1:1 care from the midwife she had hoped for. Postnatally, Izumi is very tearful and expresses her disappointment that centred on loss of control and failure to realise her birth expectations.

Key discussion points

1. In the context of perinatal mental illness what are the main risk factors identified by this scenario?
2. What actions should the midwife take?
3. What support should Izumi receive?

This scenario is a useful reminder to midwives that with appropriate support (Hodnett and Fredericks 2003, Webster et al 2000, Oakley et al 1996), women such as Izumi will be resilient enough to overcome the pain, fear and at times crippling anxiety of pregnancy, labour and birth. However, for others, traumatic events around their labour and birth experience will remain indelibly imprinted in their psyche, and may blight their lives and affect the relationship with not only their baby but also their partner. PTSD may result in the woman experiencing nightmares or 'flashbacks', which can be very distressing and frightening when the woman is again confronted with real images of labour (Lyons 1998). Although psychological interventions such as '**debriefing**' have been suggested to ameliorate immediate symptomatology, there is no reliable evidence that it is a useful intervention in reducing psychological morbidity (Bick et al 2009, Alexandra 1998). It is for this reason that NICE (2007) does not recommend routine debriefing, rather healthcare professionals such as midwives should support women who wish to talk about their experience. Neither should they overlook the impact of a traumatic birth on the partner. Major life events in general can challenge a woman's coping reserves and lead to distress, especially when social support is lacking. Scenario 4.3 is reflective of some of the major life events that can prove disruptive to women's coping abilities.

Case scenario 4.3 Significance of major life events

Melanie is a 24-year-old single/unsupported mother, expecting her third baby. At her antenatal booking she looks very anxious and informed the midwife that she and her long-term partner recently separated acrimoniously. Her mother who was her only reliable means of support died eight months ago following the impact of a road traffic accident. Melanie expresses her anxieties about the future, as the pregnancy is unplanned. She was given Prozac by her GP shortly after the death of her mother.

Key discussion points

1. What are the risk factors, if any, of a perinatal mental illness?
2. Does Melanie need perinatal psychiatric referral (justify your answer)?
3. How may the midwife respond?

The 'blues'

The postnatal 'blues' is a frequently observed phenomenon which occurs in the first week postpartum, where women are susceptible to transient tearfulness and emotional lability. It is therefore depicted as a common dysphoric, transitory and self-limiting state. It has been identified as an antecedent to depression following childbirth (Cooper and Murray 1995, Gregoire 1995) rather than a psychiatric disorder per se.

Incidence

It is experienced by 50–80% of women depending on parity (Cox and Holden 1994, Harris et al 1994).

Clinical features

The mean onset typically occurs between the third and fourth postpartum day and may last up to a week or more but rarely persisting longer than 48 hours. Features may include emotional lability (e.g. weepiness, despair, irritability to euphoria and laughter). The new mother might feel overwhelmed by the sudden realisation of the relentless responsibility of the baby's 24-hour dependency and vulnerability (Raynor 2006).

Aetiology

The actual cause is unclear though hormonal influences (changes in oestrogen, progesterone and prolactin levels) are implicated. The onset of the 'blues' seems to coincide with the production of milk in the breasts, as well as the quality of social support.

Care/management

This state of heightened emotionality is self-limiting and will resolve spontaneously, assisted by social support (Chapter 8) mainly from loved ones. Vigilance from the midwife, use of the Whooley questions (Whooley et al 1997, NICE 2006, 2007) and selective postnatal visits tailored to meet the mother's needs (Bick et al 2009, DH 2004) will help to identify persistent features that could be suggestive of depressive illness.

Prognosis

Due to the self-limiting and transient nature of the 'blues', with effective support women do regain some sense of equilibrium quickly. Arguably, as such a large percentage of women are affected by the 'blues', within a feminist paradigm it is seen as a normative process or period of transition and adaptation to change and not a mental illness (Nicholson 1998). However, the 'blues' is often cited as a precursor to depression (Cooper and Murray 1995, Gregoire 1995).

Mild postnatal depressive illness

It has been illustrated that depression after childbirth represents a kaleidoscope pattern that may take different forms. At the mildest end of the spectrum the illness may present as an exaggeration of the various emotional changes during the puerperium, which may not be easily distinguishable from the emotional upheavals associated with the transitional phase of motherhood. Mild depressive illness in the postpartum period is the commonest of all the PMIs that may present at this time.

Incidence

The reported incidence of this condition is mired in controversy and contradictions partly due to problems of definition and the diagnostic criteria used. Nonetheless it is thought to affect about 10–15% of all women postpartum (Cooper and Murray 1995, 1997b, Cox et al 1993). It is no commoner after childbirth than amongst women in the general population of childbearing age, but who are not mothers.

Risk factors

A number of risk factors have been implicated in the manifestation of mild postnatal depressive illness such as stressful life events e.g. marital discord (Beck 2001, O'Hara and Swain 1996) and lack of social support (Dennis et al 2004, Beck 2001, Cooper and Murray 1998, O'Hara and Swain 1996). The woman might have a previous history of depression or have been mildly depressed during the last trimester of pregnancy. A number of studies such as Evans et al (2001) have shown that depression in late pregnancy is as high as depression in the postpartum period. Astbury (2001) reflects that over the life span it is estimated on average women are more vulnerable to depression than men, experiencing the illness between 1.6–2.6 times more commonly than men. This difference is most transparent during the childbearing years when women are engaged in the care of young children (Oates and Raynor 2009).

Aetiology

The actual cause of mild postpartum depressive illness remains unclear with many studies suggesting numerous confounding variables, though the presence of psychosocial risk factors identified above, seem to dominate (Cooper and Murray 1997b, Cox et al 1993).

Clinical features

Although women may have difficulty getting to sleep and experience appetite difficulties, both over-eating and under-eating, the classical presentation of a biological syndrome evident in severe depression is usually not apparent. The onset is more gradual or insidious during the puerperium and more commonly presents after the first three postpartum months. Features are variable but often there is irritability, tearfulness, anxiety, ideas of not coping, self-blame, guilt and unhappiness. There may also be a sense of loneliness but these mothers' mood tend to lift when they are in company rather than alone (Oates 2006).

Mother–baby relationship

Even in the mildest form, depression following childbirth creates a vicious cycle and unwanted sequelae that may lead to a fractious mother–baby relationship (Cooper and Murray 1997a). Lack of pleasure in the baby may stem from the infant being very unsettled in the early months following birth, e.g. a baby who seems to constantly cry, is difficult to feed, comfort and settle can just as often be the cause of a mild postnatal depressive illness as the result of it. A longer period of structured postnatal visits by the midwife for women with known vulnerability factors has been recommended (Bick et al 2009, NICE 2006, DH 2004). During this time midwives should bear in mind that a very small percentage of women who suffer from mild depressive illness may experience such marked irritability or even hostility towards their baby that puts the child at risk of being injured.

Care/management

Like all the other illnesses covered in this chapter, clear guidance on the management of mild postpartum depressive illness is detailed in the full *Antenatal and Postnatal Mental Health* guidelines from NICE (2007), who recognise that a combination of psychological interventions such as listening visits provided by the health visitor and social support are superior treatment to antidepressants. The results of a recent multi-centred randomised controlled trial reported by Dennis et al (2009) concluded that telephone based peer support is a useful and efficacious intervention in the prevention of mild depressive illness in women with known risk factors. This demonstrates that the supportive role of a significant other is a crucial factor in determining health and wellbeing. Hormonal treatment such as use of progesterone therapy is not recommended (NICE 2007, Dennis et al 1998).

Prognosis

Early recognition, timely and appropriate management that considers the socio-cultural circumstances of the mother, baby and family should contribute to a swift improvement in the mother's condition within weeks and recovery by the time the infant is 6 months old. Without treatment the mother may experience prolonged psychological morbidity.

Relationship with partner

Understanding the impact of a postpartum depressive illness on the partner and family dynamics is developing (Deater-Deckard et al 1998) and continues to emerge within the literature. However, there needs to be more studies to build a critical mass of information. Factors to consider when supporting partners especially fathers are detailed in Figure 4.3.

Role of the midwife: learning lessons from key reports

The DH (2004) stresses the need for a culture where care is evidence based. There are many different types of evidence; some are more rigorous than others, but for the purpose of this section of the chapter emphasis will be placed on the *Maternity National Services Framework* (DH 2004), NICE and SIGN guidelines as well as relevant CEMACH reports. In order to reduce the effects of PMI on the woman, fetus/neonate, existing children and family, midwives have been identified as pivotal public health professionals in assessing those mothers at risk of psychiatric disorders (NICE 2008, 2007, DH 2004). Part of the midwife's role is to help prevent and reduce psychological morbidity by promoting positive maternal and paternal mental health. Strategies to achieve this must be reflected in parent education classes. Midwives need to be skilled in assessing the dynamic process involved in mother–baby interaction, and be conversant with safeguarding/child protection issues. Midwifery care in the postnatal period needs urgent review in the light of recommendations by the DH (2004), identifying that women with known vulnerability factors need psychological support and continuity of care by the midwife up to 90 days postpartum. This is even more important with early transfer home from hospital of women who have given birth in the hospital setting (Brown et al 2008). There also needs to be identified care pathways that address gaps between primary and secondary mental health care as well as education/training and learning opportunities for positive multi-agency working. Successive CEMACH reports (Lewis 2007, Lewis and Drife 2004) have highlighted the importance of good communication practice within the multidisciplinary team and interagency working. Opportunities should therefore exist to ensure effective channels of communication not only in primary care but across interagency and secondary care.

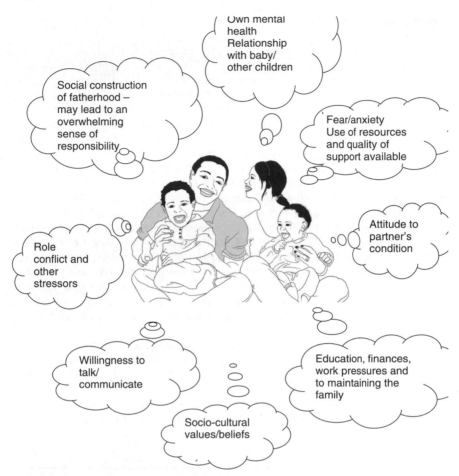

Figure 4.3 Factors to consider when supporting the partner of a mother with a postpartum depressive illness

Continuity of care with carer is also imperative. It is recommended that GPs for example, provide information during the antenatal period that is accurate, appropriate, transparent and complete. This information should account for the woman's past, current or family history of psychiatric disorders and communicated to the midwife. Midwives are now the first point of contact for many pregnant women. If effective care is to be achieved it is fundamental that during the maternity period the midwife and the GP have mutual respect for each other and foster a harmonious working relationship where information can be shared. This information sharing antenatally is crucial as it will further assist the midwife in making routine but sensitive enquiries about previous psychiatric history in a systematic way (NICE 2008, 2007, SIGN 2002). In rare cases the woman may conceal a past history of mental illness from her partner. Therefore if the partner is present, the midwife will need to find an opportunity to ask the question again without the partner being in attendance, and consider issues of safeguarding, confidentiality and record keeping. Statutory midwifery supervision can be a useful mechanism to help support both the woman and midwife. Midwives should remember that support by a mental health nurse or mental health team can be requested for women during pregnancy and postpartum, but guidelines for referral must be in place to make the process smooth and problem free.

Midwives need a firm understanding of the range of normative emotional reaction adjustments or changes around childbirth (Winson 2009). This resonates with the RCPsych (2000b) recommendations that healthcare professionals involved in caring for women with SMI within psychiatric services need the necessary knowledge and competencies to make skilled decisions. A clear understanding of the perinatal context is therefore required coupled with a familiarity with the physiological processes of pregnancy, childbirth and the emotions involved in the transition to motherhood. Like NICE (2007), the RCPsych (2000b) also states that a working knowledge of psychotropic medication in pregnancy including the distinctive clinical features of the range of PMI that present during the childbearing continuum is essential. Only then can midwives make a substantial contribution to reducing psychological morbidity by enhanced parent education classes that addresses the reality of parenthood. When screening for past, present or family history of psychiatric disorders it must be remembered that midwives are not psychiatric nurses. They will need to be educated in order to develop skills in information framing to ask valid questions that will elicit the appropriate response from pregnant women. Nationally, the kind and content of pre-registration curricula will vary in how much emphasis and time is given to topics such as PMI. Some areas have no dedicated perinatal service. Even where such facilities exist, midwives still need their knowledge base regularly updated to maintain their understanding, confidence and competence when screening for risks. Interprofessional Objective Structured Clinical Examination (ITOSCE) or 'skills and drills' training could be one way of achieving this.

As key public health workers midwives play a pivotal role in health promotion there is now a specific need for midwives to help meet government policy and targets in relation to public health issues. PMI is a major part of this policy initiative. In England NICE (2007) and in Scotland SIGN (2002) provide guidance for the specific but comprehensive range of PMI. NICE (2007) also provides details about the implications of pharmacological treatments and their implications on breastfeeding, which are outside the scope of this chapter.

Managed care networks

NICE (2007), Standard 11 of the *Maternity National Services Framework* (DH 2004) and CEMACH (Lewis and Drife 2004) highlight the importance of integrated care pathways and managed care networks (MCNs). MCNs provide a structured and integrated multidisciplinary approach to care for health professionals working in primary, secondary and tertiary centres. MCNs allow for robust care pathways to ensure that care is individualised and tailored to meet the specific needs of women with PMI at all levels as they progress through the healthcare system. Working together to improve choices for women, provide better pathways of care and promote improved use of shared resources will help provide a more appropriate and better balance of care (DH 2003b, 2004, 2007a, 2007b).

Suicide

Although PMI is a significant contributor to maternal morbidity and mortality, suicide is substantially less common in pregnant and postpartum women and often cited as a very rare occurrence indeed (Appleby et al 1998). Yet the sobering findings of successive reports into maternal deaths in the UK (Oates 2001, 2004, 2007) cite suicide as a leading cause of maternal mortality. Often accounting for 10–15% of maternal demise, deaths from psychiatric causes overall contribute to 25% of all maternal mortality (Oates 2004). Maternal suicide occurs more frequently than previously thought (Oates 2007), especially with the reporting of such deaths to ONS up to one year post-birth. Oates (2007) states that in the past such deaths were woefully underestimated and under-reported; even though the maternal suicide rate appears to be equivalent to that of the general rate in the female population, and is uncommon in pregnancy, women with SMI could be at risk.

Socio-economic factors

Looking at the trends that have emerged from the psychiatric chapter in the CEMACH reports (Oates 2001, 2004, 2007) it would appear that suicide is not correlated with socio-economic deprivation. Most cases of the suicides reported reflect women who were generally well supported, not socio-economically deprived, in stable relationships, and older; also a number of these women were health professionals. Another trend is that in most cases the suicides were violent in nature including **self-immolation**, hanging and jumping from a great height. This serves to demonstrate just how precipitous and grave SMI can be, and supportive of the need for antenatal screening.

Previous history

Another lesson to be learnt is that a significant number of the women in the Confidential Enquiries who committed suicide had a history of SMI but fell through the net at antenatal booking. Tellingly, this is detailed in the extract below (Oates 2007:160):

A young woman living in stable circumstances killed herself in a violent manner several weeks after the birth of her baby. She had previous history of bipolar illness with a number of inpatient admissions for mania. She had last been seen by psychiatric services shortly before the beginning of her pregnancy and appeared to have stopped her mood stabiliser medication at this time. Although the GP mentioned her previous psychiatric history in his referral to the obstetrician, the midwife appears to have been unaware of this at booking. The woman remained well throughout her pregnancy but no steps were taken to monitor her mental health following birth. Shortly after birth she had non-specific mental health problems resulting in an assessment by a duty psychiatrist. No steps were taken to inform her GP, midwife or health visitor nor to refer her back to psychiatric care. A few weeks after birth, she saw her GP for depression but he did not feel that she was mentally ill. The day before her death, relatives contacted the health visitor, but not the GP or psychiatric services, because of their concern about the woman.

From this case vignette it can be seen that the appropriate care pathway was not followed and no proactive management plan was mobilised. Had these processes been activated perhaps this death and others might have been avoided (Oates 2007). This is why there is such a strong emphasis for midwives to make sensitive enquiry during the antenatal period about a history of SMI (NICE 2008, 2007, DH 2004, Oates 2001).

Medical conditions caused by or mistaken for psychiatric disorder

It is clear that in some cases of maternal death physical symptoms were misattributed to psychiatric conditions. A number of deaths cited in CEMACH (Oates 2007) occurred due to physical illness that was misattributed to mental illness, and took place in a psychiatric unit. Mislabelling and misdiagnosis result in substandard care and is a serious risk manage-ment issue. As can be seen in the extract detailed below taken from a case vignette in the CEMACH report (Oates 2007: 156), it is worth remembering that a physical illness does and can complicate psychiatric disorders.

A woman died in the early weeks post-birth from a PE and aortic dissection. She had been admitted in late pregnancy with severe upper back pain, thought at the time to be musculoskeletal in origin, overlaid with anxiety. Her pain continued following birth and a few days later she was admitted with a history of breathlessness and chest pain and haemoptysis. She was agitated, frightened and thought she was dying. She was diagnosed with 'PND' and referred to a psychiatrist. He found a frightened and physically ill woman who did not have a primary psychiatric disorder. The woman died shortly afterwards.

Sharing best practice

In response to the NHS plan (DH 2000), *Making a Difference* (DH 2001) and to fulfil the remit of NICE (2007) and meet the maternity standards as delineated in the maternity National Service Framework (DH 2004), some midwives have already 'grasped the nettle' and taken on an enhanced public health role, developing specialist or link roles in the field of perinatal mental health. In England, many midwives also work within children's centres and Sure Start services. These link midwives can play a critical part in helping to meet the continuing education needs of their colleagues, helping them to use the care pathways that are in place for women at known risk of a PMI. Figure 4.4 was developed by Nottinghamshire Perinatal Mental Health Management Network Group, a group that reports to the first MCN for mental health to be established in England, located in the East Midlands Strategic Health Authority. This screening tool is instrumental in assisting midwives in detecting women at risk of SMI and making appropriate referrals. It was developed as a result of the findings from earlier Confidential Enquiries into maternal deaths in the UK (Oates 2001) and is an example of good practice.

Conclusion

PMI represents an array of psychiatric disorders that might either be pre-existing, co-exit with pregnancy or develop after childbirth. Psychiatric postpartum illnesses are relatively common, may take different forms and are sometimes predictable. All are treatable and mothers generally respond favourably to treatment and do get better. Pregnancy and the puerperium provide ample and unprecedented opportunities for screening and detection of such illnesses. This is a unique opportunity for multidisciplinary and intra-agency collaboration in both primary and secondary healthcare settings. There is now sound evidence that enduring mental illness can have a significant detrimental impact on the wellbeing of the woman, the fetus and the infant (Murray and Cooper 2003, Cooper and Murray 1997a). This is of particular concern when combined with social adversity such as poverty and social isolation. It is crucial that continuity of care and effective communication practice coupled with close liaison between key agencies are efficient and robust to support women and their families. This is in consideration of findings reported by CEMACH (Lewis 2007) that suggest that suicide, while significant, is not the only factor in maternal deaths related to psychiatric reasons. Women die from other sequelae linked to their psychiatric condition. Some of these are due to accidental overdoses from illicit drugs and from physical illness that might not have developed in the absence of a psychiatric illness. Such stark findings have major implications for the multidisciplinary team involved in the care of women with PMI. Improved communication, more dedicated perinatal mental health service and interprofessional education, plus maximising opportunities to work more closely together will help to reduce maternal morbidity, avoid care that is sub standard and ultimately prevent maternal deaths (Oates 2007).

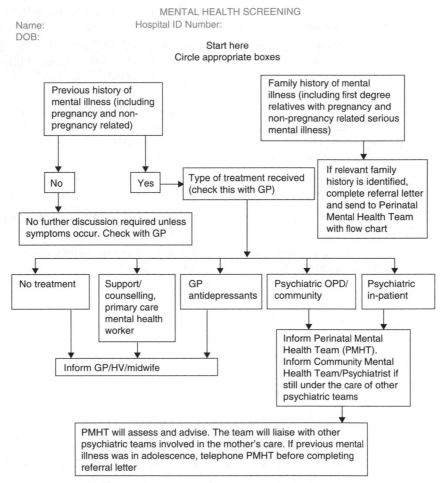

Figure 4.4 An antenatal screening tool for detecting perinatal mental illness

---

Summary of key points

- PMI is a major public health issue and a leading cause of maternal morbidity and mortality in the UK.

- Midwives must make sensitive enquiry into women's current and previous mental health at first contact i.e. antenatal 'booking' (NICE 2007, 2008; Lewis 2007, DH 2004, Lewis and Drife 2004).

- There is insufficient evidence that diverse psychosocial or psychological interventions reduce the number of women who develop a postpartum depressive illness. However, interventions that target vulnerable women and are individualised, or, initiated postnatally, are more likely to have a positive impact.

- The full range of psychiatric disorders can complicate pregnancy and the postpartum year.

- The incidence of affective disorder, particularly at the most severe end of the spectrum, increases following birth.

- The familiar features of psychiatric disorder are all present in postpartum disorders, but the early maternity context and the dominance of infant care and mother–infant relationships exert a powerful effect on the content, if not the form, of the symptomatology.

- Early maternity is a time when there is an expectation of joy, pleasure and fulfilment. Thus the presence of a psychiatric illness is particularly distressing. The midwife must therefore be a skilled member of the multidisciplinary team to provide care that is sensitive and considers the women's socio-cultural background.

- Care must involve multidisciplinary and multi-agency working, especially close relationships with maternity and children's services.

- The term 'PND' should be avoided as it undermines the severity of a mental illness (Oates 2004, 2007).

- Care/management of PMI must consider the health and wellbeing of the family especially the impact on the partner and existing children.

References

Affonso, D.D., De, A.K., Horowitz, J.A. and Mayberry, L.J. (2000) An international study exploring levels of postpartum depressive symptomatology. *Journal of psychosomatic research*, 49: 207–16.

Alexandra, J. (1998) Confusing debriefing and defusing postnatally: the need for clarity of terms, purpose and value. *Midwifery*, 14(2): 122–4.

Appleby, L., Gregoire, A., Platz, C., Martin, P. and Kumar, R. (1994) Screening women for high risk of postnatal depression. *Journal of Psychosomatic Research*, 38: 359–545.

Appleby, L., Mortenson, P.B. and Faragher, E.B. (1998) Suicide and other causes of mortality after postpartum psychiatric admission. *British Journal of Psychiatry*, 173(9): 209–11.

Astbury, J. (2001) Gender disparities in mental health. In: *World Health Organization Mental Health: a call for action*. Geneva: WHO, pp 73–92.

Barclay, L. and Lloyd, B. (1996) The misery of motherhood: alternative approaches to distress. *Midwifery*, 12(3): 136–8.

Barlow, J., Coren, E. and Stewart-Brown, S. (2002) Parent-training programmes for improving maternal psychosocial health. *Cochrane Library of Systematic Reviews*, Issue 4. Art No: CD002020. DOI: 10.1002/14651858.

Beck, C.T. (2001) Predictors of postpartum depression: an update. *Nursing Research*, 50: 275–85.

Bick, D., MacArthur, C., Knowles, H. and Winter, H. (2009) *Postnatal Care: evidence and guidelines for management*, 2nd edn. Edinburgh: Churchill Livingstone.

Brown, J., Small, R., Faber, B., Krastev, A. and Davis, P. (2008) Early postnatal discharge from hospital for healthy mothers and term infants. *Cochrane Library of Systematic Reviews*, Issue 4. Art No: CD002958. DOI: 10.1002/14651858.

Brown, J., Harding, S., Hattersley, L. and Rosato, M. (2005) Socioeonomic differentials in health: illustrations from the Office of National Statistics longitudinal study. *Health Statistics Quarterly*, 1: 5–15.

Cantwell, R. (2003) Detection and screening in perinatal psychiatry. *Psychiatry*, 2: 20–5.

Cantwell, R. and Smith, S. (2006) Prediction and prevention of perinatal mental illness. *Psychiatry*, 5(1): 15–21.

Choi, P., Henshaw, C., Baker, S. and Tree, J. (2005) Supermum, superwife, super everything: performing femininity in the transition to motherhood. *Journal of Reproduction and Infant Psychology*, 23(2): 167–80.

Cooper, P.J. and Murray, L. (1998) Postnatal depression. *British Medical Journal*, 316: 1884–6.

Cooper, P.J. and Murray, L. (1997a) Effects of postnatal depression on infant development. *Archives of Disease in Childhood*, 77: 97–101.

Cooper, P.J. and Murray, L. (1997b) Prediction, detection and treatment of postnatal depression. *Archives of Diseases in Childhood*, 77: 97–9.

Cooper, P.J. and Murray, L. (1995) The course and recurrence of postnatal depression. *British Journal of Psychiatry*, 166: 191–5.

Cox, J.L. and Holden, J.M. (1994) Translations of the Edinburgh postnatal depression scale. In: J.L. Cox, J.M. Holden (eds) *Perinatal Psychiatry: Use and Misuse of the Edinburgh Postnatal Depression Scale*. London: Gaskell, pp 248–70.

Cox, J.L., Murray, D. and Chapman, G. (1993) A controlled study of the onset, duration and prevalence of postnatal depression. *British Journal of Psychiatry*, 163: 27–31.

Cox, J.L., Holden, J.M. and Sagovsky, R. (1987) Detection of postnatal depression: development of the Edinburgh postnatal depression scale. *British Journal of Psychiatry*, 150: 782–6.

Deater-Deckard, K., Pickering, K., Dunn, J.F. and Golding, J. (1998) Family structure and depressive symptoms in men preceding and following the birth of a child. The Avon Longitudinal Study of Pregnancy and Childhood Study Team. *American Journal of Psychiatry*, 155(6): 818–23.

Dennis, C. (2005) Psychosocial and psychological interventions for prevention of postnatal depression: systematic review. *British Medical Journal*, 331(15). DOI:10.1136/bnj.331.7507.15, accessed 24 January 2009.

Dennis, C., Hodnett, E., Kenton, I. et al (2009) Effect of peer support on prevention of postnatal depression among high risk women: multisite randomized controlled trial. *British Medical Journal*, 338: a3064, DOI:101136/bmj.a3064, accessed 24 January 2009.

Dennis, C.L., Janssen, P.A. and Singer, J. (2004) Identifying women at-risk for postpartum depression in the immediate postpartum period. *Acta Psychiatric Scandinavia*, 10: 338–46.

Dennis, C.L., Ross, L.E. and Herxheimer, A. (1998) Oestrogens and progestins for preventing and treating postpartum depression. *Cochrane Database of Systematic Reviews*, Issue 3 Art No CD01690 DOI: 10.1002/114651858.CD001690.

Department of Health (2007a) *Maternity Matters: choice, access and continuity of care in a safe service*. London: DH.

Department of Health (2007b) *Our Health, our Care, our Say: making it happen – one year on – third sector*. London: DH.

Department of Health (2004) *National Service Framework for Children, Young People and Maternity Services: maternity services standard 11*. London: DH.

Department of Health (2003a) *Mainstreaming Gender and Women's Mental Health*. London: DH.

Department of Health (2003b) *Choosing the Best: choice and equity in the NHS*. London: DH.

Department of Health (2001) *Making a Difference: the nursing, midwifery and health visiting contribution – the midwifery action plan*. www.dh.gov.uk, accessed 2 February 2009.

Department of Health (2000) *The NHS Plan: a plan for investment, a plan for reform*. www.dh.gov.uk, accessed 2 February 2009.

Elliot, S. (1994) Uses and misuses of Edinburgh postnatal depression score in primary care: a comparison of models developed in health visiting. In: J.L. Cox and J.M. Holden (eds) *Perinatal Psychiatry: use and misuse of the Edinburgh postnatal depression scale*. London: Gaskell, pp 221–8.

Evans, J., Heron, J., Francomb, H., Oke, S. and Golding, J. (2001) Cohort study of depressed mood during pregnancy and childbirth. *British Medical Journal*, 323: 257–60.

Gregoire, A. (1995) Hormones and postnatal depression. *British Journal of Midwifery*, 3(2): 99–104.

Harris, B., Lovett, L. and Newcombe, R.G. (1994) Maternity blues and major endocrine changes: Cardiff puerperal mood and hormone study 2. *British Medical Journal*, 308: 949–53.

Hodnett, E.D. and Fredericks, S. (2003) Support during pregnancy for women at increased risk of low birthweight babies. *Cochrane Database of Systematic Reviews*, Issue 3. Art. No. CD000198. DOI: 10.1002/14651858.CD000198.

Jomeen, J. and Martin, C.R. (2005) Self-esteem and mental health during early pregnancy. *Clinical Effectiveness in Nursing*, 9(1–2): 92–5.

Kendell, R.E., Chalmers, J.C. and Platz, C. (1987) Epidemiology of puerperal psychoses. *British Journal of Psychiatry*, 150: 662–73.

Kumar, R. (1994) Postnatal mental illness: a transcultural perspective. *Social Psychiatry and Psychiatric Epidemiology*, 250–64.

Kumar, R. and Robson, K.M. (1984) A prospective study of emotional disorders in childbearing women. *British Journal of Psychiatry*, 144: 35–47.

Leverton, T.J. and Elliot, S.A. (2000) Is the EPDS a magic wand? A comparison of the Edinburgh postnatal depression scale and health visitor report as predictors of diagnosis on the present state examination. *Journal of Reproductive and Infant Psychology*, 18(4): 280–96.

Lewis, G. (ed.) (2007) *Saving Mothers' Lives: reviewing maternal deaths to make motherhood safer 2003–2005*. The seventh report on Confidential Enquiries into Maternal Deaths in the United Kingdom. London: CEMACH. www.cmace.org.uk.

Lewis, G. and Drife, J. (eds) (2004) *Why Mothers Die 2000–2002*. The sixth report of the Confidential Enquiries into Maternal Deaths in the United Kingdom. London: CEMACH. www.cmace.org.uk

Lewis, G. and Drife, J. (eds) (2001) *Why Mothers Die 1997–1999*. The fifth report of the Confidential Enquiries into Maternal Deaths in the United Kingdom. London: RCOG.

Lyons, S. (1998) A prospective study of post-traumatic stress symptoms 1 month following childbirth in a group of 42 first time mothers. *Journal of Reproduction and Infant Psychology*, 16: 91–105.

Murray, L. and Caruthers, A.D. (1990) The validation of the Edinburgh postnatal depression scale on a community sample. *British Journal of Psychiatry*, 157: 288–90.

Murray, L. and Cooper, P.J. (2003) The impact of postpartum depression on infant development. In: I. Goodyer (ed.) *Aetiological Mechanisms in Developmental Psychopathology*. Oxford: Oxford University Press.

Murray, D., Cox, J.L., Chapman, G. and Jones, P. (1995) Childbirth: life event or start of a long term difficulty? Further data from Stoke-on-Trent controlled study of postnatal depression. *British Journal of Psychiatry*, 166: 595–600.

National Screening Committee (2001) *Screening for Postnatal Depression*. www.nsc.nhs.uk, accessed 25 January 2009.

National Institute for Health and Clinical Excellence (2008) *Antenatal Care: routine care for the healthy pregnant women, CG 62*. www.nice.org.uk.

National Institute for Health and Clinical Excellence (2007) *Antenatal and Postnatal Mental Health: clinical management service guidance, CG45*. www.nice.org.uk.

National Institute for Health and Clinical Excellence (2006) *Postnatal Care: routine postnatal care of women and their babies, CG 37*. www.nice.org.uk.

Nicholson, P. (1998) *Postnatal Depression: psychology, science and the transition to motherhood*. London: Routledge.

Oakley, A., Hickey, D., Rajan, L. and Rigby, A. (1996) Social support in pregnancy – does it have long term effects? *Journal of Reproduction and Infant Psychology*, 14: 7–22.

Oates, M.R. (2007) Deaths from psychiatric causes. In: G. Lewis (ed.) *Saving Mothers' Lives: reviewing maternal deaths to make motherhood safer 2003–2005*. The seventh report on Confidential Enquiries into Maternal Deaths in the United Kingdom. www.cemace.org.uk.

Oates, M.R. (2006) Perinatal psychiatric syndromes: clinical features. *Psychiatry*, 5(1): 5–9.

Oates, M.R. (2004) Deaths from psychiatric causes. In: G. Lewis, J. Drife (eds) *Why Mothers Die 2000–2002: The sixth report of the Confidential Enquiries into Maternal Deaths in the United Kingdom*. www.cemace.org.uk, Chapter 11.

Oates, M.R. (2001) Deaths from psychiatric causes. In: G. Lewis, J. Drife (eds) *Why mothers die 1997–1999: The fifth report of the Confidential Enquiries into Maternal Deaths in the United Kingdom*. www.cemace.org.uk, chapter 11.

Oates, M.R. (1996) Psychiatric services for women following childbirth. *International Review of Psychiatry*, 8: 87–98.

Oates, M. and Raynor, M.D. (2009) Perinatal mental health. Part B: perinatal psychiatric disorders. In: D.M. Fraser and M.A. Cooper (eds) *Myles Textbook for Midwives*, 15th edn. Edinburgh: Churchill Livingstone, pp 686–704.

Office for National Statistics (2002) *Living in Britain, General Household Survey No 31*. London: ONS.

O'Hara, M.W. and Swain, A.M. (1996) Rates and risk of postpartum depression – a meta-analysis. *International Review of Psychiatry*, 8: 87–98.

Phoenix, A. and Woollett, A. (1991) Motherhood: social construction, politics and psychology. In:

A. Phoenix, A. Woollett, E. Lloyd (eds) *Motherhood: meanings, practices and ideologies.* London: Sage, pp 13–27.

Raynor, M. (2006) Pregnancy and the puerperium: the social and psychological context. *Psychiatry,* 5 (1): 1–4.

Robertson, E., Jones, I., Hague, S., Holder, R. and Craddock, N. (2005) Risk of puerperal and non-puerperal recurrence of illness following bipolar affective puerperal (postpartum) psychosis. *British Journal of Psychiatry,* 186(6): 258–9.

Robling, S.A., Paykel, E.S., Dunn, V.J., Abbott, R. and Katona, C. (2000) Long-term outcome of severe puerperal psychiatric illness: a 23 year follow-up study. *Psychological Medicine,* 30: 1263–71.

Royal College of Psychiatrists (2000a) *Perinatal Maternal Mental Health Services.* Report CR88. London: RCPsych.

Royal College of Psychiatrists (2000b) *Report on Recommendations for the Provision of Mental Health Services for Childbearing Women.* London: RCPsych.

Scottish Intercollegiate Guidelines Network (2002) *Postnatal Depression and Puerperal Psychosis.* SIGN Publication No.60. www.sign.ac.uk.

Ussher, J. (1992) Reproductive rhetoric and the blaming of the body. In: P. Nicholson and J. Ussher (eds) *The Psychology of Women's Health and Health Care.* Basingstoke: Macmillan, pp 13–61.

Webster, J., Linnane, J.W.J., Dibley, L.M., Hinson, J.K., Starrenburg, S.E., Roberts, J.A. (2000) Measuring social support during pregnancy: can it be simple and meaningful? *Birth,* 27(2): 97–103.

Whooley, M.A., Avins, A.L., Miranda, J. and Browner, W.S. (1997) Case-finding instruments for depression two questions are as good as many. *Journal of General Internal Medicine,* 12(7): 439–45.

Winson, N. (2009) Transition to motherhood. In: C. Squire (ed.) *The Social Context of Birth,* 2nd edn. Oxford: Radcliffe, pp 145–60.

Annotated further reading

Grabowska, C. (2009) Unhappiness after childbirth. In: C. Squire (ed.) *The Social Context of Birth,* 2nd edn. Oxford: Radcliffe Press, Ch 14, pp 236–50.

A useful chapter that provides food for thought around some of the factors that may lead to unhappiness following childbirth.

The Children's Act 2004. www.opsi.gov.uk/acts2004, accessed 21 January 2009. Updated Act – provides guidance on legal issues relating to child protection.

To explore the impact of depressive illness on the partner and family dynamics the reader should access and read the following:

Ramchandani, P., Stein, A., Evans, J. and O'Connor, T.G. (2005) Paternal depression in the postnatal period and child development: a prospective population study. *Lancet,* 365(9478): 2201–5.

Schumacher, M., Zubaran, C. and White, G. (2008) Bringing birth-related paternal depression to the for. *Women Birth,* 21(2): 65–70. www.ncbi.nlm.nih.gov/pubmed, accessed 21 January 2009.

Tammentie, T. (2004) Family dynamics and postnatal depression. *Journal of Psychiatric and Mental Health Nursing,* 11: 141–9.

A useful article.

World Health Organization (2009) *Mental Health Aspects of Reproductive Health: a global review of the literature.* www.who.int, accessed 1 February 2009.

Useful websites

Birth Trauma Association: www.birthtraumaassociation.org.uk
Fathers Direct: www.fathersdirect.com
Fatherhood Institute: www.fatherhoodinstitute.org
Perinatal Illness UK: www.pni-uk.com

5 | The psychology of communication in midwifery practice

Chapter contents

Introduction

Chapter aims

The psychology of communication: the holistic approach

Building the working alliance: the rapport

The psychology of the first impression

Beyond first impressions: the psychology of building a relationship

Qualities of the midwife as an effective communicator

Relating in depth with other people – does it happen?

Assertiveness: the key to successful communication

The humanistic approach to communication

Listening and attending: the essential communication skills for woman-centred care

Listening, presence and touch

Barriers, constraints and difficulties that influence effective communication

Conclusion

Summary of key points

References

Annotated further reading

Introduction

Effective communication is a caring skill like any other skill that is learned and perfected. However, the factors that influence the use of communication skills are invariably changing. Most people tend to develop their own personal and professional repertoire of communication skills that they perceive work for them and this is monitored by their self-awareness, which in itself can be enhanced or reduced by situational variables. Hence the process is complex and subjective. When communication is done really well, its processes can go relatively unnoticed but the benefits derived from its presence are felt and enjoyed by everyone involved. Done badly, any sense of personal worth can be threatened, tarnished or irreparably damaged. It is widely accepted that effective high quality communication between midwives, their clients and their families is vital in enhancing feelings of value and wellbeing (Donnelly and Neville 2008). This enables mothers to become active partners in decision-making. Positive communication between professionals creates a cohesive atmosphere and leads to more coordinated care. Kindness, respect and understanding are the hallmarks of interpersonal cooperation, and communication skills are the glue that holds it all together (Nursing and Midwifery Council (NMC) 2008, Royal College of Obstetricians and Gynaecologists (RCOG) 2008).

This chapter will explore the psychology of communication in a holistic way and show how different situations and elements influence the way people respond and interact with others. It will include the psychology of how first and subsequent impressions can affect the different ways a professional rapport is established. It will draw upon the counselling theory of Carl Rogers and apply his core conditions of empathic understanding, unconditional positive regard and congruence because they are recognised 'ways of being a certain kind of person' that frames the midwife's attitude into making the mother's care truly 'person-centred', a philosophy that is more likely to cherish childbirth as a satisfying, valued experience, rather than a distressing event that may diminish her.

Chapter aims

- To discuss communication messages sent verbally, vocally and via the body

- To explore the psychology of establishing and maintaining a rapport in holistic communication

- To explore the psychology of making first and subsequent impressions

- To support the view that empathic understanding, congruence (genuineness) and unconditional positive regard (acceptance and warmth) are attitudes that enable the midwife to be an effective communicator

- To stress the importance of developing assertiveness skills in being an effective communicator with mothers and colleagues alike

- To emphasise that quality communication may mean that the midwife offers presence, stillness, silence and when appropriate touch

- To be aware of barriers to effective communication

The psychology of communication: the holistic approach

Performing a physical task skilfully is not enough. Donnelly and Neville (2008) assert that effective communication is *imperative* in providing high quality care and has a direct impact on how that care is perceived (Kitzinger 2009). Midwives need to be able to effectively communicate with the people they are attempting to help. Childbearing women have many complex needs that are not purely physical and practical but are also psychological and spiritual. They may need help in coping with feelings, handling distress, managing change and finding words to express themselves. There is also the most important need of being understood. Wright (2007) believes that most mothers manage to communicate well, but others may be in pain or discomfort, are frustrated, sad or disadvantaged. Others may not speak the same language or have words with which the midwife is familiar. Communication is not simply about words but *how* they are said, transmitted and received (see Case vignette 5.1).

Box 5.1 The different dimensions of communication

A. Verbal messages sent via words. Words can have a powerful effect on people as they can inform, inspire, make them laugh and cry, induce fear and anxiety.

- Language can be formal/informal, based in colloquialisms or expressions may be indigenous to the local area, referred to as the vernacular

- Use of excessive abbreviations and professional jargon pose the greatest risk to verbal expression as midwives and their multi-agency and professional teams become blinkered to their use and are often totally bemused by their client's look of confusion and bewilderment when they ask for further explanation (Riley 2008)
- Schott et al (2007) assert that euphemisms such as 'passed away' when used instead of the words died and death, are not helpful. Describing a person as 'gone' invites the response 'gone where?'
- Linguistic diversity is the norm with over 300 languages being spoken in the United Kingdom (Gill et al 2009). Gestures and sign language help but by far, interpreting services enhance client satisfaction (Thom 2008)
- Content of talk may focus on oneself, others or neutral issues. May have an evaluative dimension whether positive and upbeat or negative e.g. 'I feel happy about the pregnancy but fearful of the test results'
- Ownership of speech where 'I' and 'you' words emphasise the focus
- Amount of speech. Some people are extremely talkative; some talk a lot but say little, others offer little, but say what they need to

B. Vocal messages sent through the voice sometimes referred to as paralanguage.

- Tone and volume refers to loudness and softness. A firm and confident voice that can be easily heard is desirable. A booming voice overwhelms. Soft voices are comforting and reduce tension but may imply non-assertiveness in certain circumstances (See Chapter 7 for further discussion on tone)
- Rate refers to the amount of words used in a specific time and the pauses between them. If delivered too quickly, understanding may be lost through fatigue, but the faster a person speaks, the more competent they may appear (Nelson-Jones 2009). When too slow and ponderous, speech may become boring. The use of appropriate silence is an important aspect of speech rate. If there are no words to say, it is better to remain silent. Silence is often misinterpreted but never misquoted. If the midwife is imparting significant news the rate is slower than usual to enhance clarity and understanding
- Clarity refers to the ability to enunciate words. The words are expressed in an articulate way and mumbling is avoided. Trailing off at the end of a sentence, stuttering and over-repetitious use of habitual words like 'you know' interfere with flow and concentration
- Pitch refers to the height or depth of the voice. An anxious person tends to pitch too high and the timbre (the quality) is often strained. The female midwife when imparting significant news may lower her pitch to complement a soft tone and slower rate of expression. This approach helps understanding when the recipient perceives the information as bad news (Bryant 2008)
- Emphasis on certain words to cause effect, but must be appropriate as too much can sound melodramatic; too little, flat and wooden

C. Messages sent by the body (body language or non-verbal communication).

- Facial expressions. According to Glasper and Quiddington (2009), learned from an early age, the smile is probably the only international language shared by people everywhere (See Chapter 7). There are six recognised facial expressions of emotion and these are happiness, disgust, fear, sadness, surprise and anger. The hundreds of other facial expressions seen are derived from these and are therefore sometimes difficult to interpret
- Gaze is a way of looking at a person without staring and for not too long. Argyle (1999) asserts that women are more visually attentive than men in all measures of gaze. More time is spent in gazing at speakers compared to listeners

- Eye contact is looking at the other person's eyes and is related to gaze. This is a very cultural-specific activity and can be perceived as intrusive even offensive for some people, but essential for others (Orr and Morris 2009)
- Posture relates to turning the body to or away from the other person. Height is associated with status so sitting may eliminate the talking 'up to' or 'down to' scenario (Nelson-Jones 2009)
- Appearance mediated through appropriate clothes and grooming will define a person in terms of social and occupational standing
- Chronoemics is the way people react to time and can lead to agitation and anxiety (Peate 2006)
- Olfactrics is the study of smell (and associated memories). It can cause people to relate or disengage according to factors such as a fragrance or poor personal hygiene
- Proxemics is the distance people maintain while communicating with others. This can range from 2 to 12 foot, dependent upon the nature of the relationship (intimate/social) and contextual activities. Personal space may be invaded by touch and may include hand shaking, hugging and kissing, but there is wide cultural variation and caution is the key word
- Kinetics is communicating through facial or bodily movements like head nodding, raising eyebrows, hand gestures.

Building the working alliance: the rapport

Within every midwife, there is the person within the role. These two aspects of the person are not easily separated, but the person may emerge in more intimate, supportive, facilitative interactions with the role counterpart being seen more as the professional, more authoritative individual. Whatever the circumstances this means, at its most basic level, the midwife shows an interest in the mother as a fellow human being.

Case vignette 5.1

Irene has been waiting for over half an hour to see the midwife. This is her first pregnancy. She is 44 years of age and feels anxious about the booking appointment. Norma the midwife has had a busy booking clinic, she is running late and it is now 17.00hrs. She invites Irene into the room and apologises for keeping her waiting. Norma is acutely aware of her fatigue but knows that she must listen to Irene with a keen ear and eye, offer an open attitude and suspend any preconceived ideas or judgements about her. She needs to concentrate on what Irene is saying, what she is asking for and what she needs, with no sense of hurry. Norma introduces herself and clearly explains the purpose of the booking appointment.

Norma's approach emphasises Irene's individuality. Active listening, validating and encouraging are communication skills that build a connection or emotional bond, which goes beyond a simple interaction between two people. Rapport can be seen as pacing and leading. The midwife metaphorically walks alongside the mother, pacing together, with the mother determining 'the direction in which to walk'. By pacing and building rapport over the first few minutes of a meeting the midwife builds a sense of trust in which the mother, at an unconscious level, feels safe and valued. This is referred to as emotional pacing. Other types of pacing include language pacing. By really listening *to the way* the client is using language, the midwife can pick up cues that offer insight into how she is sensing at the time. According to Pinel (2006), the main representational systems are auditory, visual, and kinaesthetic. A person functioning in an auditory sensing way may use words like 'I hear what you say' or 'it sounds good'. They will sometimes cue the listener by flicking their eyes from side to side. By comparison, a visual communication may be 'I see what you mean' or 'the future looks good' and may gaze upwards to see something in their 'minds eye'. Kinaesthetic or touch sensing may be represented as 'I feel excited' or 'I feel really scared' and looking down may indicate they are feeling something or are having an internal dialogue with themselves. A rapport is for some people an instant connection that is perceived by both as something special and enduring. For most it is a process that builds over time and is often dependent upon first impressions.

The psychology of the first impression

Meeting people for the first time in the antenatal/postnatal clinic, labour or antenatal/postnatal ward, or the woman's own home will have its different pressures given the activities that occur in these locations. Smith and Mackie (2007) believe that the raw materials of first impressions are the way people look and how they act. These cues are informative only because it is thought that *appearance and behaviour* reflect personality characteristics, preferences and lifestyles. The midwife's uniform has the effect of diminishing personal characteristics with a strong indicator of role but personal grooming and adornments will contribute to the image that the midwife will create and the mother may respond to.

The impact of communication on the first impression

According to Mehrabian (1971) up to 70% of a person's total communication is at the non-verbal level, is extremely important and not easily faked. The tone of the voice makes up around 35% of the communication and only 7% is the actual verbal content. Non-verbal responses tend to appear before the verbal ones and minimal changes in facial muscle tone can alert the receiver to the crucial parts of what a person is saying (see Box 5.1). Impressions made from non-verbal communications are subconsciously attended to and are enduring. Mehrabian (1972) believes that people who readily express their feelings non-verbally are more liked than non-expressive individuals. Members of Western cultures tend to like people who orientate their bodies towards the person they are addressing, face them directly, lean towards them and nod while speaking. This behaviour indicates that the person likes the other. Dilated pupils are also a sign of interest and attention. Such non-verbal communication offers special insight into people's moods and emotions. In Germany, Hong Kong, Japan and the United States, people express sadness and happiness, fear and anger, surprise and disgust with similar body postures and facial expressions and they interpret them in similar ways, thus supporting the view that emotional expression is a kind of universal language. However, recent findings show interpretations of emotional expressions often differ between Western and non-Western cultures particularly in emotions of surprise, sadness and disgust (Bierhoff 2008).

Case vignette 5.1 continued

Norma notices as the booking interview proceeds, that Irene is playing with her wedding ring and fiddling with her jacket. She looks uneasy and clearly is anxious and preoccupied. Norma gently poses the question 'I'm sensing from you Irene, that you are concerned about something . . . would you like to tell me what it is?' Irene looks at Norma, hesitates, then asks her whether she thinks she is too old to have a baby.

Non-verbal leakage

According to Oliver and Endersby (1994), people are leaking their true feelings and thoughts when physical responses convey a different message from their words being used. This may indicate that the person is uncomfortable or is not being totally truthful and attempting to hide something. Alternatively the person may be confused or anxious. Non-verbal leakage may present as repetitive leg swinging when seated, hair stroking, an unusually high-pitched tone of voice, a nervous laugh. The person exhibiting these behaviours is often unaware of them. The recipient of non-verbal leakage may feel uneasy as they have detected cues, usually subconsciously, that do not match with the words spoken. The midwife needs to remember that the face is more easily controlled and the body is where most people leak their intention. There may be times when the midwife herself unintentionally leaks her own representations of thoughts and feelings.

First impressions taken from physical appearance

There is an assumption that the way people look is usually the first cue to what they are like. Hassin and Trope (2000) argue that impressions based on people's appearance can alter interpretations of what they say. Physical attractiveness, particularly the face, calls up a variety of positive expectations. It is assumed that what is highly attractive is good and such people are more intelligent, interesting, warm, outgoing and socially skilled compared to less attractive people, and for this reason is an important element in people's attraction to strangers. A person who has a familiar look generally leads to increased liking by another (Smith and Mackie 2007). Unusual or salient characteristics capture attention and are regarded as not only making a difference in creating impressions of others, but also help to define oneself, because what is unusual to one person may be of little importance to another.

Two crucial kinds of *stored knowledge* help the person to interpret perceived cues

1. Associations already learned. Associations link two cognitive representations and if either of the linked associations is triggered, the other will usually appear too. For example, Fiona's demeanour reminds the midwife of her aunt who is totally unreliable. The midwife may then unwittingly perceive Fiona as unreliable. Members of different cultures have different associations and therefore arrive at different interpretations for the same behaviour.

2. Thoughts that are currently in one's mind. Current thoughts may activate cognitive representations making them highly accessible and likely to affect interpretations. Also the mood of the person may colour their interpretation. For example, a person in a cheerful mood is more likely to make a more positive favourable impression than one who is tired, anxious or in a hurry. A reminder from an object or event may colour the impression too.

People often assume that others have inner qualities that correspond to their observable behaviours. The *correspondence bias* (the fundamental attribution error) is made when people interpret the way another acts and believe this reflects their inner qualities rather than the effects of *situational pressures*. In Western cultures, individuals are seen as independent and autonomous, responsible for their own thoughts, feelings and actions. It follows that Western observers tend to assume that people's inner dispositions cause their behaviours. In non-Western cultures, people are assumed to be *interdependent with*, rather than *interdependent from*, groups. Thus, situational as well as personal factors are used when explaining behaviour (Choi et al 2003). This factor is worth considering when working with or caring for people from different cultures.

Beyond first impressions: the psychology of building a relationship

Parkinson (2008) argues that to go beyond first impressions the midwife needs to be sufficiently motivated to do so and have enough opportunity to thoroughly assess the mother, which will require adequate time to think with freedom from distractions. When situational factors (and not the person's disposition) appear to have caused a particular behaviour, the perceiver may attempt to correct an initial inference but this correction takes time and sometimes does not occur. All the typical demands of everyday interaction like trying to remember other people's names and faces, planning what to say next or working to give a good impression, require considerable cognitive energy. The midwife's impressions may be very much at the mercy of the behaviours she happens to see the mother perform first.

Once an impression has been formed, rather than conducting an unbiased search for accuracy, people look for evidence that supports their preferred conclusions. Most of the time people are blind to their own biases as they think what they see is actually what is, because they consider they can construct a coherent representation of reality. However, when comparing their view with those of others, their own biases may become more apparent. Any attempts at correction will depend on the midwife's beliefs about the nature and direction of the bias. Thus the primacy effect first described by Asch in 1946 allows for information presented earlier being more influential than that presented later (Parkinson 2008). Motives and expectations slant judgements. Once a person has formed an impression of another person, their expectations often lead them to behave in ways that elicit expectation-confirming behaviours from others. The skill is to work from the mother's agenda and make no assumptions. Sheldon (2005) believes that communication occurs on two levels, the relationship and content level. The relationship level refers to how the two participants are bound to each other. The content level is the use of words, language and information. The two levels are inextricably bound because content is relayed more effectively in healthy relationships. In strained relationships the message is likely to be corrupted because the person is struggling with the relationship.

Case vignette 5.1 continued

Norma reassured Irene that her situation is not unusual and offered her evidence-based information concerning the number of women having their first pregnancy at an older age. Irene appeared comforted by how and what she was told. Norma remained quiet to enable Irene to assimilate the information and when Irene resumed eye contact with her, Norma asked 'Are you ready to continue?'

When Irene's age was raised as a concern, Norma could have simultaneously introduced antenatal screening for fetal abnormality. Although a logical approach from the midwife's perspective, this could have presented Irene with yet another dilemma. Norma decided to finish the information collecting part of the interview and introduce the topic of antenatal screening later. According to Parkinson (2008), a person's vulnerability to shaping by others' expectations will depend upon the person's uncertainty of their views of self, their poor awareness of the views others have of them and their social motives in the situation. The need for Irene to 'get on with her midwife' may render her compliant and ready to conform to anything Norma implicitly or explicitly expresses. Midwives are often unaware of their organisational and knowledge power and the influence they may have on mothers and their families (see Box 5.2). The social pressure that exists in the midwife–mother role partnership may inhibit the mother from informing the midwife of what she desires; therefore the onus is on the midwife to build a rapport where a persuasive communication style is *not* utilised (DH 2007). When antenatal screening was discussed, Irene confidently told Norma that she knew what choices were available and had decided to opt out. Norma accepted her decision and made an appropriate entry on to her file. It would have been so easy for Norma to make the assumption that as an older mother, Irene's greatest fear was of having a baby with a congenital abnormality, not her uncertainty of motherhood itself.

Goodall et al (2009) found in their study of how communications affected decision-making in mothers' birth choice following caesarean section (CS) that mothers were not well enough informed to make a decision because medical practitioners used a non-specific, indirect communication style. They offered choice but then expressed personal opinions about the success rate of the options available without identifying reasons. They adopted a latent style of persuasive communication, which appeared explicit, but was laden with prophecies of 'you will probably end up with a CS'. This type of communication has a (not so) hidden agenda, but effectively disables choice as it appears to be offering a choice while simultaneously inhibiting the mother in her decision-making processes (see Box 5.2).

Box 5.2 Persuasive communications. Factors that may contribute to persuading another person to act in a particular way.

Reflect upon how you obtain consent from a mother for an intervention.

The midwife as source:

- his/her status and credibility
- physical attractiveness
- trustworthiness
- use of congruent non-verbal communication

How the message is delivered:

- the consistency of the non-verbal communication-the absence of non-verbal leakage
- tone of voice
- whether it is an explicit or implicit message
- its level of emotional appeal
- balanced arguments that offer all aspects of the issue
- the order of presentation (consider primacy effect)
- a crisp and well-timed summary

The mother as recipient:

- her level of education and knowledge base
- her attitudes to health care, its providers, motherhood etc.
- her resistance to persuasion based on previous experiences
- her level of apprehension, anxiety, confusion.

Qualities of the midwife as an effective communicator

From the humanistic perspective, Mearns and Thorne (2007) believe that to be an effective communicator, the midwife must be expressive enough as a person to communicate in an unambiguous way, to be perceived by the other person as trustworthy, dependable and consistent, in some deep sense and to express positive attitudes of warmth, caring, liking, interest and respect. Schott et al (2007) endorse this view and believe it is also important to free the other person from the sense of being judged, by accepting, when presented, each aspect of them. This may mean their tears, anger, even a sense of weakness. The midwife needs to act with sufficient sensitivity in the relationship so as not to be perceived as a threat. However, the midwife should feel strong enough to be separate from the other person and to be secure enough to permit this separateness (Rogers 1961). On this last point, take for example the parents who receive life-changing news. Their baby has a major congenital abnormality. The midwife through caring for this family, by association, may feel in some way responsible, but as Bryant (2008) believes, this is not an uncommon reaction, but is irrational thinking, often triggered by witnessing the anguish of the people involved. Midwives are able to help people to cope with overwhelming sadness and disappointment but it is easy to become drawn into their grief. This sense of separateness must prevail, to safeguard their self-concept and mental health (see Chapter 7).

Some midwives believe that clinical practice does not allow for such intimacy to take place. They imply that this type of closeness takes time to develop. This is a misconception often held by midwives who have little experience of working with, or being close to, mothers and their families. They may have had poor outcomes in working with vulnerable people or hold the view that it is not their job to 'provide a shoulder to cry on'. Some relationships only last for a few minutes, some a few hours or days, others span months. A therapeutic relationship is health-focused and woman-centred with defined boundaries. Its purpose is to support and enhance psychological and physical functioning (Sheldon 2005).

Relating in depth with other people – does it happen?

Mearns (1996) argues that most of human relating does not take place at depth and this is perhaps why people place great value on it when they experience it themselves or hear about it from others. It is seen as a rarity. Are people too afraid of others or of themselves, or both, to risk meeting each other at relational depth? Like hedgehogs, do people want to be close enough to feel each other's warmth, but not too close that they can feel the prickles? Mearns (1996) further asserts that people relate to each other through a screen, likened to a lace curtain which allows a degree of permeability which for some acts as an illusion that there is some depth-relating going on. The screen for others needs to be virtually impermeable, should experiencing the problems of others hurt them too much. Sometimes the screen becomes a habit, for example the false smile. This smile does not reflect an inner feeling of warmth or appreciation but exists as a defence to pre-empt even the possibility of any negativity in the other's response. Over-effusiveness and politeness are other habitual screens. An effective psychological communication does not always take place at a deep level. There will be superficial and other levels of contact that are perfectly normal and a functional part of human relating. The crucial element is that the midwife is willing to move to deeper levels, if the woman or colleague is willing and able (Schott et al 2007).

Assertiveness: the key to successful communication

To be assertive is to have the ability to express one's thoughts, ideas and feelings without undue anxiety, without expense to others. The assertive midwife appears confident, comfortable, caring, non-judgemental and clear. The assertive mother tends to be well informed, have a need to be heard, be involved in decision-making and will not want to be dependent upon the 'expert' (DH 2007). Some mothers are not assertive and may adopt aggressive or passive communication styles. See Case vignette 5.2.

Case vignette 5.2

Lucy is in labour but progress is slow. She is fault finding, argumentative and uncooperative. She requires extensive explanations, reassurance and encouragement. She is perceived as demanding by her midwife who is harbouring feelings of irritation, impatience and frustration towards her as she is affecting the midwife's ability to cope with the other mothers in her care. The midwife feels afraid of being trapped by a complainer and perceives her as an attention-seeker. Lucy's care becomes fragmented, as her frequent calls for attention are not always heeded. If Lucy and her midwife's expectations are at odds, or when fresh demands on the relationship cannot be negotiated, it may come to a dysfunctional and regrettable standstill.

When there is perceived difficulty, there is a strong temptation to put as much distance between oneself and the other person. This is a common mistake when working with women, their families and colleagues because it nurtures the psychological void. Sometimes the assertive response is to listen for more information. Lucy clearly needs more, not less attention. The midwife needs to understand the cause of her behaviour (see Box 5.3). The midwife should ask her manager in an assertive manner to re-allocate some of her work. She should then consider her own attitudes towards Lucy and attempt to reconcile any difficulties with her. Sustained contact and continuity offer a more successful and satisfying outcome.

Reflective activity 5.1

In your day-to-day practice, how would you manage this situation?

How do you respond to the notion of asking for some of your work to be reallocated?

- always do
- should do so more often
- is a waste of time

Are there other responses that you have thought about?

Balzer-Riley (2008) argues that assertive communication skills make interactions more equal. All parties have a right to express their thoughts, feelings and beliefs. Assertive behaviour is a life-long learning skill that requires time and practice, but is a matter of choice. With each person encountered in any situation, there is a choice whether to communicate assertively, aggressively or passively. The words chosen and how they are expressed will influence the outcome, and realistically people do not always have the energy or desire to exert their rights on every occasion. There are times when people cannot respond rationally, such as when they are worried, over-tired or anxious. The timing, content and receptivity of the recipient will affect the effectiveness of the communication. If Lucy were not English speaking, consider the difficulties in attempting to help her and how this might adversely affect morbidity and mortality outcomes (Schenker et al 2008, Lewis 2007).

Box 5.3 Personal language

People protect their vulnerability through defence mechanisms (see Chapter 1) and this may be expressed through the use of personal language. Instead of becoming judgemental about the mother's behaviour, the midwife may ask 'what does this behaviour mean for this mother?'

- Mary's tears means she is angry
- *That* smile from Zabina means she is hurting
- Sarah's laughter means she is tense or embarrassed
- Laura's irritability may mean she is scared and in pain
- Lynne's repeated lateness probably means she is uneasy about what is happening
- Laura's quietness means she doesn't understand.

The midwife may need to explore with the mother what she is attempting to hide or convey.

The humanistic approach to communication

Rogers (1980) asserts that the mother is the expert on herself and with this knowledge the midwife needs to be able to communicate positive attitudes to her, to find some common ground on which to establish authentic dialogue. A combination of unconditional positive regard (acceptance, warmth), congruence (genuineness) and above all empathic understanding will help the midwife to create a mutual partnership and empower the mother to value herself and her contributions to her childbearing experiences (Kitzinger 2009). Rogers (1980) argues that these attitudes cannot be packaged into techniques or strategies, but are part of the midwife's own innate and learned communication style.

The attitude of unconditional positive regard (acceptance, warmth)

For a midwife to hold an attitude towards the mother of unconditional positive regard is to accept her totally as a person, to include her strengths, weaknesses and all that she is. By comparison, conditional positive regard is how the midwife judges the mother in accordance to the midwife's own conditions of acceptance of having a relationship with the mother. The mother may only receive positive regard if she is able to bargain with the midwife what she needs to do, to fulfil the midwife's conditions.

Acceptance does not mean approval. Approval is a judgement, which can serve to disadvantage a person, and therefore is undesirable. Respect can be communicated by a welcoming attitude, by introducing oneself and asking the mother what she likes to be called. The provision of comfort and privacy is basic and fundamental. By ensuring that informed consent is comprehensively obtained for clinical interventions serves to value the mother. Any off-hand gesture or utterance can seriously undermine the relationship and set the scene for future encounters.

Warmth is a feature of a relaxed person and is especially communicated in the voice by quiet soft modulated tones. Speech cannot be pressured, stilted or stoic and the pacing should be in keeping with the speaker's natural breathing. It is only possible to express warmth when one has a genuine interest in the other person and a wish to convey that feeling to them. A desire to be warm is based on the belief that each person encountered is worthy of receiving the acceptance and comfort that one's warmth generates. When midwives display high-level warmth they are completely and intensively attentive to the interaction between themselves and their clients or colleagues, making them feel accepted and important.

The opposite is cool behaviour, which conveys disapproval or uninterest. Thoughts and feelings that act to distract one's attention from other people block the expression of warmth. Being rushed, being overcome by strong emotions or being judgemental are classic distractions. When one feels hurt, bitter or simply irritated with a mother or colleague, attempting to convey warmth would be insincere. At times one may hide behind a crisp façade when feeling insecure about whether one will be rejected or accepted by another person, although façades tend to leave the other person feeling confused. Only when one feels secure in the relationship, will warmth surface again. Sometimes the midwife may have strong negative feelings towards someone who has complained to them or about them, or treated them with coldness, disdain or even rudeness and contempt. When one wants to protect oneself from perceived or actual uncaring or disinterest, one may withdraw warmth or refrain from offering it. According to Balzer-Riley (2008), it is assertive to express warmth to others when one wishes. It is passive to withhold the warmth felt and it is aggressive to exude warmth beyond the measure of one's feelings. When one sincerely conveys the warmth felt, one expresses 'I like myself, I like you'. This warmth is non-possessive and enables others to be themselves. Nelson-Jones (2009) notes that acceptance of another person involves compassion for human frailty and an understanding of the conditions that lead people to behave in a less than desirable way. Rejecting a person for their human failings is not helpful in restoring their self-worth to cope with their present life situation.

Reflective activity 5.2

It is said that one person's warmth may be perceived as another person's patronage or sentimentality. A patron is a protector, a supporter, but patronage behaviour is sometimes communicated in a condescending way.

What feelings are aroused as a result of being patronised?

What can be learned from this experience in communicating with others?

The attitude of congruence (genuineness)

It is acknowledged that warmth can be difficult to convey without patronising the mother and this is why Raskin et al (2008) assert that it is so closely linked to congruence or being genuine. To be genuine is to present one's thoughts and feelings (one's awareness), both verbally and non-verbally in a consistent, transparent way to another person. How the words are said, the facial expressions and body posture, all contribute to the overall communication. It is the real picture that conveys an individual's experience, not a distorted image that differs from how one really is (see Box 5.3). It does not mean to impulsively off-load one's reactions on to others. To do this is to behave aggressively. In a therapeutic relationship, presenting one's thoughts and feelings to others can be done assertively and constructively. See Case vignette 5.3.

Case vignette 5.3

Helen, a junior student midwife assisted Ruth to birth her baby and was now drying baby Joseph in preparation for his skin-to-skin contact with her. Helen noticed that Joseph had positional talipes equinovarus and quietly informed her mentor. At that point Ruth's partner John asked if everything was all right with his son. The midwife handed Joseph back to Ruth and responded to both parents by saying that Joseph's right foot had been squashed while in the womb and was slightly out of alignment. As she spoke she demonstrated to them how easy it was to bring the foot back into its correct position. Ruth asked if 'this deformity' was her fault. The midwife explained that the small amount of amniotic fluid that surrounded Joseph in the womb may have contributed to this condition, but was emphatic that there was not anything that Ruth could have done to change the situation. John then asked whether Joseph was likely to have any other problems. The midwife told the couple that she would perform a thorough examination of Joseph, to screen for any other defects.

This is not an easy situation for the midwife, but she was able to tell the parents her professional opinion and what needed to be done. Rogers (1980) asserts that being authentic and transparent translates into self-confidence. In its absence, the midwife may find it easier to tell the parents what she thinks they want to hear, in an effort to spare their feelings and feel accepted and important. This is paternalistic behaviour and is not treating the parents as adults. Even though Ruth and John are distressed by the information they have received, success when measuring a communication skill, is the midwife's ability to connect at a level that is meaningful to the people involved. This includes Helen, who is part of this interaction. The different roles that midwives assume have cultural, gender and situational performance expectations. Being genuine means remembering that roles are created by individuals with unique personalities, styles and ideas. Realness means being relatively free from the conceptual boundaries of the role and not hiding behind the façade of the role. Being a person and a midwife at the same time involves spontaneity as one cannot act from a preconceived script or get it right every time (Nelson-Jones 2008).

Reflective activity 5.3 A comment from Jo, an experienced midwife

'. . . occasionally when I hear what I have just said, I feel embarrassed because the words have come out wrong or the tone was too harsh . . . immediately I apologise and correct it. Parents are very forgiving . . . and it's as if they accept my mistake and are more accepting of me.'

The attitude of empathic understanding

Natural empathy is a basic human endowment and is an important part of the use of self but many people choose not to use it in their everyday encounters with people because it involves listening skills and they prefer to talk. Some feel they are not empathic. It is an intrinsic ability to understand the feelings of others but is arguably different to clinical empathy, that is a skill deliberately employed to achieve a therapeutic intervention (Williamson 2008). It is not the attitude of empathy by itself that is beneficial, but the intention of the giver and the perception of the receiver. Not all midwives offer an empathic way of being. Rogers (1980) argues that empathy has the highest priority of the attitudinal elements of communications in promoting relationships. When mothers or colleagues are hurting, confused, troubled, anxious, or doubtful of self-worth, then understanding is called for. Empathy dissolves alienation and can contribute to feelings of increased self-esteem on the part of those to whom one extends it.

When empathising with a mother, there is an initial need to listen carefully and seek to put oneself in her place, followed by making an emotional shift from thinking to feeling. This is when the midwife stands metaphorically side by side with the mother in a heartfelt understanding about the experience just shared. Balzer-Riley (2008) argues that when the midwife's self-identity, personal values and boundaries develop, it is easier to retain one's own identity in interactions with mothers and thus feel one with others, without prejudice. She goes on to say that the highest level of empathy is when one recognises the other's humanity and personhood regardless of any ambiguous circumstances. According to Rogers (1980) empathy is communicating understanding. To fully understand without judging, the midwife does not question why the mother reacts in a certain way or tells her to feel differently.

The combining influences of unconditional positive regard, congruence and empathetic understanding

The three attitudes and their related skills are the drivers of effective communication (Rogers 1980). However, it is easy to get it wrong and on some occasions diminished warmth will speak louder than any words of empathy and the mixed message of caring words and uncaring gestures may lead to confusion and resentment (Mearns and Thorne 2007). See Case vignette 5.4.

Case vignette 5.4

Robbie has been a midwife for 35 years. She is seen as the person who expertly orders the stock and does the off-duty. Her approach to care is mostly task-orientated and her contact with mothers and their families is usually superficial with excessive talking, usually about trivia. She is a kind person. Her communication style has evolved over the past few years.

This type of communication style serves a minor social function but is often a coping mechanism for those who wish to distance themselves from emotionally needy people (Mearns and Thorne 2007). By not fully utilising her empathy skills and offering warmth in her role, she communicates a desire for non-involvement that in time could contribute to a loss in job satisfaction. Poor assertiveness skills and perceived low self-esteem may contribute to her poor listening ability.

Listening and attending: the essential communication skills for woman-centred care

Listening can be a difficult skill to acquire because it takes time and sometimes midwives are so concerned about giving information (and advice) that they are unable to see the advantage of enabling the mother to make her own decisions. Bertram (2008) believes that when a midwife gives a mother advice, she is saying that she knows better and when she insists on doing something to solve the mother's problem, she has psychologically failed her (Egan 2007). This is not woman-centred care, it is midwife-centred and usually makes the midwife feel better and in control but may contribute to the mother's sense of fear and weakness. The mother if nurtured can do it for herself. She is not helpless. When the midwife listens and accepts that the mother feels the way she does, even though it sounds irrational, the mother can then work on the source of her feelings (Bertram 2008).

According to Balzer-Riley (2008) there is a *yearning* to be understood and it feels good to be listened to and means that the mother is taken seriously; her ideas and feelings are known and ultimately what she has to say matters. Poor listeners, who smile and nod with a vacant look or are posed to jump into the conversation with the next part of *their* text, are not listeners but talkers and rapidly inhibit the person who *needs* to talk (see Box 5.4). To be an effective listener is a most challenging skill to acquire as many people think that being quiet for a moment, taking their turn in a conversation, is listening. This is perhaps more hearing what is being said but not taking into account the whole person; the words being used, the way the words are being emphasised and the person's body language (see Box 5.1). Listening is not a passive activity and requires considerable cognitive energy and in terms of concentration ability is time-limited to about 20 minutes.

The midwife must maintain eye contact without staring. She must not interrupt the talker's verbal flow and if so, only to clarify a point of understanding by paraphrasing or reflecting upon what has been covered already. The listener needs to be able to pay attention, to be still, be fully present moment to moment without trying to change anything. She need to consciously set aside her own distractions, knowing that if one is distracted, it is saying that something else is more important than the mother she is with. Her lack of concentration may be communicated non-verbally and this will undermine her efforts in attempting to be a good listener.

Reflective activity 5.4

With a colleague, ask him/her to tell you about their favourite film or holiday. Once they have started to talk, *continually* interrupt them. When they stop talking, ask the person how they felt as a result of your interruptions.

Reflective activity 5.5

With another colleague, ask them about a topic of interest to them. Once they begin to speak, offer no eye contact. Notice how long the interaction lasts. The tendency for it to fizzle out prematurely is very common in Western cultures.

Listening, presence and touch

Balzer-Riley (2008) believes that caring conversations make a difference to care plans and job satisfaction. To be present is to bear witness to the mother's experience, to understand her perspective and respect her rights to dignity and self-determination. Midwives need to also appreciate that many mothers are complete in this moment in time and do not need to be 'fixed' or made whole again. This presence or 'being with' is in contrast to 'doing to'. In times of great difficulty when words become redundant, Schott et al (2007) argue that there is an acknowledgement of kinship that is derived from a shared human experience. See Case vignette 5.5. Midwives sometimes respond to offers of thanks with 'but I didn't do anything?' From the mother's perspective they did a tremendous amount because they offered their presence and time, which is a powerful form of psychosocial support.

Case vignette 5.5

When Rose was born she did not cry and was taken to the resuscitaire. Extra help was summoned and a midwife, a stranger to parents Paul and Ellie, came into the birthing room. She introduced herself and remained with them while the multi-professional team performed the

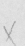

resuscitation. She explained that they would not initially hear any crying as a mask was over Rose's face. She answered questions as they arose, but most of the time she remained quiet but ready to respond. Paul was transfixed in stress and was motionless. The midwife offered Ellie touch by asking her if she would like her hand held. Ellie eagerly accepted and took Paul's hand too. There they remained, until Rose took her first breath and made initial attempts to cry.

Offering a presence with appropriate quietness, silence, soft-toned speech and clear, simple explanations is an example of excellent communication care. The midwife was a stranger to the parents but she was able to interact with them effectively because of the context and situation. Continuity of care is seen as the ideal (NMC 2008) but sometimes a professional stranger can offer a world of advantages to those in need.

Touching is a natural and literal reaching out of one person towards another, but some people find it enormously difficult to show and receive support through touch. According to Mearns and Thorne (2007) it is a circular problem because when there is not much touching it begins to be feared, mistrusted and little used. When working with mothers or colleagues the midwife needs to be aware of her touch behaviour, knowing that it should be a caring response rather than an imposition of one's own needs. To hug a person may be a midwife's way of offering comfort but the recipient may not desire this massive invasion of their personal space. The very act of touching can render a rational articulate person who is telling their story, into an upset, distressed one. Asking permission to touch a person sounds rather formal but for many midwives this strategy works because it reflects a polite and empathic attitude. Nelson-Jones (2009) asserts that touch communication must include consideration of which part of the body the midwife uses, which part of the other person's body gets touched and how gentle or firm is the touching.

Box 5.4 Barriers to effective communications. Factors that impact on the quality of communications between the people involved.

Barriers are a two way process. Poor communication by the sender will affect the message and the receiver and vice versa. Each barrier could apply to the midwife and/or the mother.

- Faking by putting on a good show of listening by nodding and giving verbal cues, but not listening at all
- Interrupting by constantly breaking in while the other is talking
- Waiting for one's turn to talk, gathering one's thoughts together then cutting others short
- Lying in wait for factual errors, then immediately correcting these errors in the other's remarks
- Criticising by passing judgement on the other person while he or she is talking. It could be criticism of their voice, mannerisms, appearance
- Failing to have knowledge/skills/confidence to provide accurate, truthful and balanced information to enable the mother to make decisions and give consent to interventions
- Lack skills in questioning, paraphrasing and reflecting skills to check for meaning and understanding
- Do not acknowledge and compensate for differences in status and perceived levels of education
- The presence of exploitation and/or harassment
- Fail to protect the mother's dignity and privacy
- Environmental odours, noise and distractions
- Disruption from other family members

- Physical, cognitive or sensory disabilities in the mother and/or family members
- Aggressive or threatening behaviour elicited by the mother or family members
- Passivity – 'can't be bothered' attitude, showing boredom and disinterest
- Maternal disorientation from administered medication(s)
- Emotional overload and denial. Feelings of sadness, tiredness, despair
- Time constraints
- Mothers and their families who cannot speak or write English
- Bigotry and prejudice. Judging others by their appearance, colour, creed, character and behaviour
- The mother who is constantly talking on her mobile phone (Orr and Morris 2009)
- Constant interruptions by members of the multi-professional team
- Inappropriate use of touch.

How do you think you communicate when you are stressed, sad, in a hurry, happy?

Apply these cognitive/emotional states to the above communication barriers and question how your behaviour may be affected.

Barriers, constraints and difficulties that influence effective communication

There is no doubt that effective communication between mothers, their families, the midwife and her multi-professional team is complex and there will be occasions when things go wrong (see Box 5.4). People adopt their own personal communication style that supports their self-concept; some feel the need to rely upon manipulative self-serving styles that tend to distance people. Satir (1988) believes they limit a person's potential for personal growth and cooperative satisfying relationships. They can promote fear and dependency in others.

Recognised communication styles that can lead to harm

- *Placating* is where a person talks in an ingratiating way to the extent that they never disagree with the other person and are constantly apologising.
- *Blaming* is dictating and acting in a superior manner, with endless fault finding and putting the fault on others.
- A *computing* style is cool, calm and collected, always correct and very reasonable, but with no semblance of feeling.
- *Distracting* as a communication style is not responding to the point but instead doing and saying whatever is irrelevant.

As Satir (1988) comments, these styles of responding do more than interfere with open and honest communication: they can also reinforce the recipient's feeling of low self-esteem. Rendering a person less than what they can be is an attempt to create a sense of superiority over them. Schafer (2000) argues that many people are *distress provokers*, sometimes intentionally and with full awareness and others quite unintentionally through poor skill development.

Each midwife in viewing her own communication style as a whole, may pose the difficult question as to whether she unwittingly acts to add stress and lessen self-worth in others? If one is engaging in communication that is not having a desirable positive effect, close scrutiny of the style adopted may indicate why. Negativity can cause or add to distress for others and through the same feedback loop is distressing for the communicator. Distress-provoking actions may include adopting and maintaining a sour facial expression, monopolising the conversation, endlessly complaining, making people feel guilty and ridiculing others. Schafer (2000) believes that offering positivity prevents distress for others and is enhancing for the giver. Rewarding communications include listening attentively, affirming the feelings and needs of others and treating others as equals whenever possible. How people interact with each other can contribute to how stressed they feel and may affect how teams work together which could have major implications for care outcomes (NMC 2008, Lewis 2007).

Conclusion

Whenever two or more people are together communication is taking place. Even in total silence and the complete absence of overt non-verbal signals, information is being transmitted as each person infers something from the other's behaviour. In social situations therefore it is impossible not to communicate. Midwives need to be able to build a rapport with a mother relatively quickly and effectively in order to provide care that is physically and psychologically intimate. There is a requirement to be attentive and to share information that is clear, accurate and meaningful, at a level that the mother and her family can understand. Midwives work in teams and the need to consult and explore ways of maximising care is essential and calls for assertive and advocacy skills in communication. Barriers to communication can range from the irritations of a busy, noisy environment to something much more pervasive such as a negative attitude that can humiliate, frustrate and ultimately spoil a life event of great significance. Such experiences are remembered and can lead to poor psychological health and recovery (RCOG 2008). Donnelly and Neville (2008) assert that when recipients of care do not feel cared for, the most common factor is the psychology of communication, expressed simply as 'how they were spoken to'. It goes to the core of the person and represents the biggest daily challenge to midwives and the teams in which they work, to get it right.

Summary of key points

- The midwife must hold a belief that effective communication is at the heart of good care.

- Creating a positive first impression should be uppermost in the midwife's thinking.

- A combination of warmth, genuineness and empathic understanding are the hallmarks of communicating a desire to connect with another person in a spiritual way that is supportive to both the giver and receiver.

- Listening skills should be developed, honed and perceived as the most useful in the communication toolkit.

- Assertiveness skills assist in working with mothers, their families and colleagues to facilitate better care but also can help protect the midwife's own self-concept and esteem.

- Barriers to communication are always present but awareness of how they can influence the behaviour of the mother, her family and the midwife is part of an ongoing vigilant process in reducing their effects.

References

Argyle, M. (1999) *The Psychology of Interpersonal Behaviour*, 5th edn. London: Penguin Books.

Asch, S.E. (1946) Forming impressions of personality. In: E.R. Smith and D.M. Mackie (2007) *Social Psychology*, 3rd edn. Hove: Psychological Press, p 85.

Balzer-Riley, J. (2008) *Communications in Nursing*, 6th edn. St. Louis: Mosby Elsevier.

Bertram, L. (2008) *Supporting Postnatal Women into Motherhood*. Oxford: Radcliffe.

Bierhoff, H.W. (2008) Prosocial behaviour. In: M. Hewstone, W. Stroebe, K. Jonas (eds) *Introduction to Social Psychology. A European perspective*. London: Blackwell, pp 176–95.

Bryant, L. (2008) Breaking bad news. *Practice Nurse*, 35(5): 37–42.

Choi, I., Dalal, R., Kim-Prieto, C. and Park, H. (2003) Culture and judgement of causal relevance. *Journal of Personality and Social Psychology*, 84: 46–59.

Department of Health (2007) *Maternity Matters*. London: DH.

Donnelly, E. and Neville, L. (2008) *Communication and Interpersonal Skills*. Exeter: Reflect Press.

Egan, G. (2007) *The Skilled Helper: a problem management and opportunity development approach to helping*, 8th edn. New York: Brooks/Cole.

Gill, D., Shankar, A., Quirke, T. and Freemantle, N. (2009) *Access to Interpreting Services in England: secondary analysis on national data*. Http://www.biomedcentral.com/1471-2458/9/.

Glasper, A. and Quiddington, J. (2009) Communication. In: A. Glasper, G. McEwing, J. Richardson (eds) *Foundation Studies for Caring*. London: Palgrave Macmillan, pp 79–93.

Goodall, K.E., McVittie, C. and Magill, M. (2009) Birth choice following primary Caesarean section: mothers' perceptions of the influence of health care professionals on decision making. *Journal of Reproductive and Infant Psychology*, 27(1): 4–14.

Hassin, R. and Trope, Y. (2000) Facing faces: studies of the cognitive aspects of physiognomy. *Journal of Personality and Social Psychology*, 78: 837–52.

Kitzinger, S. (2009) *Birth Crisis*, 2nd edn. London: Routledge.

Lewis, G. (ed.) (2007) *Saving Mothers' Lives: reviewing maternal deaths to make motherhood safer 2003–2005*. The seventh report on Confidential Enquiries into Maternal Deaths in the United Kingdom. London. CEMACH.

Mearns, D. (1996) Working at relational depth with clients in person-centred therapy. *Counselling*, Nov. 306–11.

Mearns, D. and Thorne, B. (2007) *Person-centred Counselling in Action*. London: Sage.

Mehrabian, A. (1972) *Nonverbal Communication*. Chicago: Aldine.

Mehrabian, A. (1971) *Silent Witness*. Belmont, CA: Wadsworth.

Nelson-Jones, R. (2009) *Introduction to Counselling Skills. Text and activities*, 3rd edn. London: Sage.

Nelson-Jones, R. (2008) *Basic Counselling Skills: a helper's manual*, 2nd edn. London: Sage.

Nursing and Midwifery Council (2008) *The Code. Standards of conduct, performance and ethics for nurses and midwives*. London: NMC.

Oliver, R. and Endersby, C. (1994) *Teaching and Assessing Nurses*. London: Baillière Tindall.

Orr, J. and Morris, D. (2009) Communication. In: A. Glasper, G. McEwing, J. Richardson, M. Weaver (eds) *Foundation Skills for Caring*. London: Palgrave Macmillan, pp 17–27.

Parkinson, B. (2008) Social perception and attribution. In: M. Hewstone, W. Stroebe, K. Jonas (eds) *Introduction to Social Psychology a European Perspective*. Oxford: Blackwell, pp 42–65.

Peate, I. (2006) *Becoming a Nurse in the 21st century*. Chichester: John Wiley and Sons.

Pinel, J.P.J. (2006) *Biopsychology*, 6th edn. Boston: Pearson.

Raskin, N.J., Rogers, C.R. and Witty, M.C. (2008) Client-centred therapy. In: R.J. Corsini, D. Wedding (eds) *Current Psychotherapies*, 8th edn. Belmont, CA: Thomson Brooks/Cole, pp 178–90.

Riley, J.B. (2008) *Communication in Nursing*, 6th edn. St. Louis: Mosby Elsevier.

Rogers, C. (1980) *A Way of Being*. Boston: Houghton Mifflin.

Rogers, C. (1961) *On Becoming a Person*. Boston: Houghton Mifflin.

Royal College of Obstetricians and Gynaecologists (2008) *Standards for Maternity Care. Report of a working party*. London: RCOG Press.

Satir, V. (1988) *The New People Making*. Mountain View, CA: Science and Behaviour Books.

Schafer, W. (2000) *Stress Management for Wellness*. Belmont, California, United States: Thomson Wadsworth.

Schenker, Y., Lo, B., Ettinger, K. and Fernandez, A. (2008) Navigating language barriers under difficult circumstances. *Annals of Internal Medicine*, 149: 264–9.

Schott, J., Henley, A. and Kohner, N. (2007) *Pregnancy Loss and the Death of a Baby: guidelines for professions*, 3rd edn. London: Stillbirth and Neonatal Death Society.

Sheldon, L.K. (2005) *Communication for Nurses. Talking with Patients*. Boston: Jones and Bartlett.

Smith, E.R. and Mackie, D.M. (2007) *Social Psychology*, 3rd edn. Hove: Psychological Press.

Thom, N. (2008) Using telephone interpreters to communicate with patients. *Nursing Times*, 104(46): 28–9.

Williamson, A. (2008) *Brief Psychological Interventions in Practice*. Chichester: John Wiley and Sons.

Wright, B. (2007) *Interpersonal Skills*. Keswick: M & K Ltd.

Annotated further reading

O'Cathain, A., Walters, S.J., Nicholl, J.P., Thomas, K.J. and Kirkham, M. (2002) Use of evidence based leaflets to promote informed choice in maternity care: randomised controlled trial in everyday practice. *British Medical Journal*, 324: 643–646.

A useful article in highlighting the importance of effective communication in maternity care.

Puthussery, S., Twamley, K., Harding, S., Mirsky, J., Baron, M. and Macfarlane, A. (2008) 'They're more like ordinary stroppy British women': attitudes and expectations of maternity care professionals to UK-born ethnic minority women. *Journal of Health Services Research and Policy*, 13(4): 195–201.

Highlights how racial stereotypes and cultural prejudices can affect communication with women from diverse ethnicities.

6 The birth environment

Chapter contents

Introduction

Chapter aims

Critical appraisal of the evidence

Emotional work

Perception of pain: psychological factors

Conclusion

Summary of key points

References

Annotated further reading

Useful websites

Introduction

Many factors affect women's choice and satisfaction levels in maternity care; satisfaction is often used as a critical measure of health outcomes (Goodman et al 2004). The birth environment is one such factor that has a powerful effect on how a woman feels as a person, her perception of choice and control in decision-making and her feelings of satisfaction with the overall birth experience (Hatem et al 2008, Hodnett et al 2005, Redshaw et al 2007, Green et al 1998). The birth environment is important in all cultures as reflected by the World Health Organization (WHO 1999). A Scandinavian study, for example, reports that the trend towards hospital births in Norway has seen a significant shift from home to large, impersonal, centralised maternity units, without any convincing scientific basis, bringing about a marked change in attitude and policies towards the birth environment for the Norwegians (Blaaka and Schauer 2008). This has resulted in a steep rise or drift towards interventions and the over-medicalisation of childbirth, mirroring the current position in the United Kingdom (UK). The majority of births in the UK no longer takes place in the private domain – home – but now mainly occurs in large public arenas – medically managed hospitals, despite great efforts to redress the balance.

Over half a million women give birth in England and Wales annually (Office of National Statistics (ONS) 2008), with the majority of births occurring in hospitals. Admitting women in normal physiological labour to intensively driven, high-technology consultant-led units needs further debate, contend Stockhill (2007) and Savage (2007). Not least because it raises fundamental questions about what real choice, control and satisfaction women have over decision-making and the whole philosophy of childbirth. This chapter will explore the ways in which such an approach might undermine and devalue women's experience rather than enhance it or indeed empower women to feel victorious on utilising their internal powers to birth their babies. The importance of caring for women in an environment that is convivial and conducive to progress during labour will be examined. Verity's story will be embedded as an exemplar for good practice, highlighting the birth environment as a place that enriches a woman's experience of childbirth as well as contributes to her emotional wellbeing and overall psychological health during her journey to motherhood. Consideration will also be given to how midwives can influence the dynamics of the birth environment.

Chapter aims

- To explore the evidence around hospital versus home as the place of birth

- To identify the psychological benefits of creating a family-centred and woman-centred environment for labour and birth

- To examine how the frame of reference employed by the midwife can either result in a spontaneous human birth or a highly medicalised technocratic experience for women

- To discuss the psychological dimensions of the birth environment as a contributor to a woman's perception of pain and control

---

Critical appraisal of the evidence

In the UK the evidence to support the move from home to hospital as the main environment for birth is lacking, resulting in an expensive and rather intrusive medical model of care (Tracy and Tracy 2003). The UK is not isolated in its position, as globally, the safety of the place of birth tends to be based on outcomes for mothers and babies, measured by maternal and perinatal morbidity and mortality rates (de Jonge et al 2009, Mori et al 2008, WHO 1999, Chamberlain et al 1997, Campbell and Macfarlane 1994). The WHO (1999) practical guide on normal birth emphasises the key principle of care as being able to achieve a healthy outcome for mother and baby using the minimum of interventions compatible with safety. However, in the absence of no universal definition for the term 'normal birth', WHO (1999) defines it as commencing at term, spontaneous in onset, low-risk at the start and without any deviation from normality throughout the labour and birthing process. The baby is born in a vertex presentation and both mother and baby are in good condition following birth. This perspective implies that there must be unequivocal evidence and a valid reason to interfere or intervene with what is essentially a natural physiological process. In order to have a full appreciation and under-standing of the evidence base to help women and their partners make informed choices and decisions regarding their preferred birth environment, two contrasting case vignettes are presented (see Case scenarios 6.1 and 6.2).

Case scenario 6.1 Choosing home as the right environment for birth

Megan and Jaan are in their early 40s and are expecting their third child. Lila is the couple's first child, born at home 12 years ago. Isaac who is 7 years old is their second offspring. He was born following an elective caesarean section for a breech presentation. Megan and Jaan are planning a home birth, and have employed an independent midwife.

Case scenario 6.2 Choosing hospital as the right environment for birth

Yolande and Stephen are expecting their second child. They are both 36 years old and own their own upholstery business, which they operate from home. Their 8-year-old son, Jack, was an undiagnosed breech and unplanned home birth that psychologically left Stephen feeling traumatised. Yolande would like to have her second baby at home but Stephen is more circumspect and less supportive of the idea. He voiced his concern that the thought of another home birth has reawakened feelings of anxiety as the midwife who attended Jack's birth panicked and became flustered when she realised the presentation was breech. Although the midwife who was first on the scene did not demonstrate confidence in her own abilities to assist a vaginal breech birth, the second midwife was highly skilled and very capable, taking the lead upon her arrival, reinstalling calm and gaining the couple's trust and confidence.

Reflective activity

1. From your observations and reflection on practice is the information regarding the place of birth framed in such a way that it enables women to make informed choice/decisions?
2. When discussing the birth plan with both couples featured in the case vignettes, what factors should the midwife explore about the place of birth to help them make an informed decision?
3. How may the midwife best support the couples in their quest for a home birth?
4. What support is available in your area to assist women in making informed decisions regarding the place of birth?
5. Where can the midwife receive support and inspiration when dealing with uncertainties or complex/challenging situations such as a planned home birth when there are known risk factors?

Evidence presented on the place of birth, especially home births, often creates polemic or polarised views influenced by a particular perspective and philosophy around the whole process of birth. It is difficult to comprehend why a woman undergoing a physiological process, where there are no known risk factors, should encounter obstacles in exercising her choice to birth her baby at home. Werkmeister et al (2008) state the importance of having a standard definition of normality for labour and birth, as it empowers women and midwives to use reliable data to make comparisons between the safety of home versus hospital as the optimal environment for birth. Reflecting on how data from the Mori et al (2008) study has been received and reported in the media, including esteemed peer reviewed journals such as the editorial comments of Steer (2008), Downe et al (2008) and Walsh and Downe (2008) write contentiously of the sometimes skewed reporting of data from scientific studies. This is also echoed in the critical appraisal and response by Gyte et al (2009), who state that the work by Mori et al (2008) that was supposedly subjected to rigorous peer review ahead of publication, failed to contribute to existing evidence about the safety of home birth. The impact of misinterpretation and misrepresentation of data has been consistently reported and highlighted (Page 2006, Young et al 2000, Olsen and Jewell 1998, Campbell and Macfarlane 1994). Not all published scientific reports are produced with rigorous and meticulous attention to detail. Midwives should therefore be skilled to appraise the research evidence critically as findings at times can be misleading. It is always good practice to interrogate published reports in order to uncover gaps, deficiencies and loopholes.

Biases in reporting seem to favour hospital over home as the preferred environment for birth in terms of safety. This is despite there being emerging evidence to demonstrate that planned home births can be safely achieved when facilitated by skilled midwives and robust clinical guidelines (de Jonge et al 2009, Janssen et al 2009, Johnson and Daviss 2005). Viewpoints that are inflexible and based on equivocal evidence are indefensible and cannot be substantiated.

Albeit there are different types of evidence, some rated more highly than others, randomised controlled trials for example are seen as the gold standard for clinical studies. However, women's experiences and voices are equally if not more important (Sakala et al 2006). A number of studies have emerged to provide an international perspective on the place of birth (de Jonge et al 2009, Janssen et al 2009, Johnson and Daviss 2005, Olsen and Jewell 1998) but robust evidence that is pertinent and specific to the UK is still lacking.

Walsh and Downe (2008) acknowledge the challenges in trying to adopt a neutral position when there are social biases that affect the individual practitioner's practice, values and beliefs system. Equally, their counter-argument is a valid one in that authoritative knowledge or how the evidence is viewed, interpreted and weighted is pivotal. They argue that knowledge is power and has implications for how information is framed, clinical guidelines formulated and how policy is developed. The assumption that hospital is the safest place for a woman to birth her baby is flawed, but the fact that the home birth rate in the UK average around 3% proves that credence is still being given to that maxim. Despite regional variations such as Torbay that boasts a home birth rate about ten times the national average, there is still a lot of work to be done to review the organisation of care and to support midwives in their effort to buck this trend.

The UK government have been strongly supportive of women's choice and the drive for home birth to become more accessible and available, making it more of a reality for women (DH 2004, 2007, Welsh Assembly Government (WAG) 2005). In England, *Maternity Matters* (DH 2007) has made a number of choice guarantees, with the expectation at the time of writing that they would be implemented by all National Health Service (NHS) Trusts, responsible for the provision of maternity care. The report states that women will be able to have an informed choice about the birth environment, and depending on their circumstances, they and their partners will be able to choose from one of the following three options:

- home birth
- birth in a local facility, including hospital setting (e.g. birth-centre or midwife-led unit) where the woman is under the care of a skilled midwife
- birth in a hospital setting where there is an interdisciplinary approach to the provision of maternity care/effective team work provided by midwives, obstetricians, anaesthetists and paediatricians/neonatologists because for some women this will be the safest option.

However, putting words into action can be a real challenge as demonstrated in Wales, where clear targets were set to achieve a 10% home birth rate by 2007 (WAG 2005). The deadline for implementation has now passed and this target has not been accomplished. The reality is without an increase in the number of midwives, coupled with a major shift in the culture of maternity care provision and organisational structure in the NHS in the UK, such an emboldened vision might remain a pipe dream.

In most developed countries, the Netherlands being a great exception, the home birth rate has remained fairly static at around 1%. This includes not only the UK but other European countries such as France and Belgium. This seems to be the picture in most developed Western countries, and the USA appears to be demonstrating the grip that medicalisation has had over the decades in influencing women's choice and decision-making (de Jonge et al 2009). Such stark statistics beg the question: are women given a real choice or is choice an illusory concept for the majority? This might be the case in the UK but in the Netherlands the infrastructure supports real choice for women as the results of a recent home birth study conducted by de Jonge et al (2009) proved a watershed in providing sound evidence regarding the safety of planned home births. The study proves there is no difference in maternal and perinatal morbidity/ mortality rates with planned home births compared to those in the hospital setting.

Arguably the empirical evidence provided by de Jonge et al (2009) is neither generalisable nor transferable to the UK as the Dutch system of organising maternity care is different to that in the UK. Nonetheless, it is a significant scientific study regarding the safety of planned home births, and the largest study of its kind carried out to date. The sample size involved a nation-wide cohort of 529,688 women. This research was conducted after harsh statistics emerged in the Netherlands that they had one of the highest perinatal mortality rates in Europe. The inference that home births could be a major factor for such poor perinatal outcomes could not be ignored since Dutch women have a real choice of whether to have their baby at home or hospital, with a third choosing home birth. Many individuals and groups committed to women having a genuine choice will be heartened that results of the study showed that the initial fears were ill-founded and unsubstantiated. Providing an objective, rational and well reasoned response through sound empirical evidence goes some way towards silencing the critics of home birth.

The situation in the UK is more complex; nationally, more home birth studies are needed to help to strengthen current UK policies and build a critical mass of evidence on the safety of planned home births versus planned hospital births. At the time of writing the results of the 'Birthplace in England' study by the National Perinatal Epidemiology Unit (NPEU 2008) in Oxford, was awaited. This major prospective cohort study funded by the DH in England and the National Institute for Health Research Service Delivery Organisation (NIHRSDO) programme, aims to examine the outcomes of births in different settings by comparing clinical outcomes for:

- 17,000 planned home births
- 10,000 planned births in midwife-led units
- 30,000 births in obstetric-led units.

The research also seeks answers to specific questions relating to safety, quality of care and how the provision of maternity care impacts on women's experience and satisfaction levels. Full details of the research protocol for 'National Evaluation Safety and Cost Effectiveness of Planned Place of Birth' are accessible at http://www.npeu.ox.ac.uk/birthplace. Hopefully the findings will provide much needed objective data to break the impasse and help make a difference by contributing to progressive changes in maternity care.

Emotional work

Psychologically, the birth environment, whether it is home or hospital, involves a lot of emotional work for both the mother and midwife claims Hunter (2006, 2009). Page (2006) questions whether the ideal birth environment exists but concludes that home provides a more conducive environment for a non-interventionalist and medicalised birth (see Verity's story). She also states that although creating a home-like environment in the hospital setting is no substitute for a home birth, midwives should strive to ensure that they work in a woman-centred way. Women choose to birth their babies in the setting of their choice for a variety of reasons, and unlike the home environment, hospitals are places that can be quite impersonal and disruptive for women and their families. Hospitals are places where midwives and doctors tend to dominate, and where Sandin-Bojö and Kvist (2008) suggest care in labour is more influenced by attitudes, habit and dictum rather than scientific wisdom. This may lead to unnecessary tension, stress and anxiety and pit women against the very women who are their professional carers – midwives. Hunter (2009) notes that competing and conflicting models of care can create undue worry or mental anguish that may result in 'emotion work' for women and midwives. This she defines as work undertaken to manage feelings, which is necessary in order to demonstrate congruence between emotions and behaviour. In other words the manner

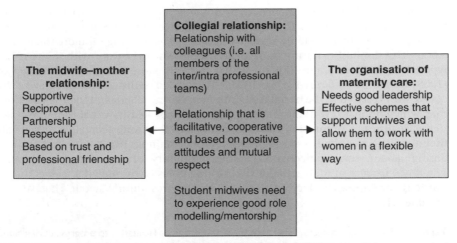

Figure 6.1 Sources of emotion work in midwifery practice (Hunter 2009)

in which a midwife or student midwife behaves or acts, based on their emotions or feelings, states Hunter (2009), must be appropriate to the given situation. Hunter (2009) and Kirkham (2000) highlight that the attitude portrayed by staff are factors in the process of communication and interpersonal relationships. Communication (see Chapter 5) is a recurrent theme in recent satisfaction surveys conducted with childbearing women (Healthcare Commission (HCC) 2008, Redshaw et al 2007). Hunter (2009) identifies three main themes or sources of 'emotion work' in midwifery practice as delineated in Figure 6.1.

Power and powerlessness

Hodnett et al (2007) report that environmental factors inherent within a hospital setting may lead to a power imbalance in the relationship between the woman and her professional carers. This may take different forms, more commonly the woman may have to relinquish control over her own body and over decision-making. Instead of feeling safe and protected in labour and birth, her baby being supported by a midwife she knows and trusts, as depicted by Verity's story, the woman may find that the competing demands and priorities on the midwife's time tend to frustrate rather than harmonise her feelings, rendering her powerless in an alien environment. This may lead to unnecessary stress, the culmination of fear and anxiety as well as increased 'emotion work' for the woman and midwife (Hunter 2006, 2009). Furthermore, Hodnett et al (2007) acknowledge the constraints and demands on midwives working in modern hospital settings by suggesting that harsh and restrictive practice may be the result of hospital rituals and routines. Such practices might prove disempowering for both women and midwives. Kirkham (1999) and Stapleton et al (2002) also highlight the power imbalance within the NHS culture that oppresses not only women but also midwives, such as the power differentials that often exist in the midwife–doctor relationship (see Chapter 2).

Use of technology – psychological effects

Births in hospitals have brought about technological advances with many births becoming a technical rather than a human experience. Technology such as electronic fetal monitoring and regional analgesia/anaesthesia i.e. epidurals, have added to intensive surveillance of labour and birth. The professional responsibilities of the midwife to attend to technology and complete endless records is now very much the norm in many maternity units, which all add to the pressure of work and stress experienced by not only the labouring woman but also the midwife (Blaaka and Schauer 2008). The shortage of midwives in the UK means that many midwives working in the NHS have to do a lot of juggling between caring for more than one woman in labour. This diminishes the opportunity for the midwife to be truly 'with woman'. In England a report by the Care Quality Commissioner, formerly known as the Healthcare Commission (2008) *Towards Better Births*, is a benchmark. It provided clarity of women's views on the quality of care they received in the hospital environment during labour and their satisfaction with that care, which resonated with the findings of the survey by Redshaw et al (2007). Women reported to the Healthcare Commission (2008) that although they were generally satisfied with the care they received, they had concerns about levels of staffing, being left alone for long periods during labour, staff competence/training, continuity of care and poor communication. The Royal College of Midwives (RCM 2008) identifies environmental factors that may prove restrictive and those conducive or facilitative of progress during labour. These are summarised in Table 6.1.

Table 6.1 Environmental factors that may prove restrictive or facilitative to progress during labour

Restrictive factors	Facilitative factors
Blanket approach to care where the woman's views, beliefs and cultural practices are ignored or not considered.	Woman-centred approach to care that is individualised and respectful of the woman's socio-cultural background, values and beliefs i.e. the heterogeneity of women is valued and respected.
Care that is undignified, unresponsive or fails to respect or be sensitive to the woman's wishes/feelings.	Care that is respectful, responsive, dignified, nurturing and sensitively considers the woman's wishes/feelings (see Verity's story).
Midwife or other health professional caring for the woman who is visibly stressed, callous and harsh and does not give the woman confidence in his/her abilities.	Midwife or other health professional that is competent, kind and empathetic. Takes time to listen to the woman and contributes towards the woman's feelings of safety, confidence and sense of relaxation.
Lack of privacy and dignity.	Woman's privacy respected and care is provided in a dignified manner.
Harsh lights.	Dimmed lights.
Clinical birthing room where bed and technology dominate. Woman more likely to be confined to the bed and have her movements restricted with limited or no access to readily available alternatives such as birthing ball, cushions and other comfort measures.	Birthing room where technology and bed does not dominate. Woman has freedom to use birthing ball, poles (other props), birthing pool, bath, shower, rocking chair, birth mats, cushions, pillows and other comfort measures.
Restrictive policies/lack of evidence base guidelines e.g. eating and drinking in labour.	Woman actively encouraged to eat and drink/willingness of midwives to meet woman's hydration and nutritive needs.
No partnership working with evident power imbalance and paternalistic approach to care.	Partnership working with diffusion of power in the mother–midwife relationship.
The woman may find herself on a collision course with her professional carers as her autonomy may be overlooked or not respected. The woman may find her views pitted against those of the midwife caring for her as well as other members of staff.	Respect for autonomy and woman's active participation in decision-making.
The environment may disempower midwives who may then find it challenging to act as women's advocates.	Midwife able to act as woman's advocate.

Medicalisation

Medicalisation of childbirth has been written about in various genres such as midwifery studies, feminism and social anthropology. All seem to draw the same conclusion that medicalisation, while it benefits the small minority of women who need it, there is a high price to pay for the blanket approach to the use of technology in childbirth, which can have deleterious effects for mother and baby (van Teijlingen et al 2004, Tracy and Tracy 2003, Kirkham 2000, WHO 1999, Tew 1998, Crompton 1996). Medicalisation has resulted in two competing and contrasting models of childbirth: the social model and the medical model. The social model views pregnancy, labour and birth as not only a biophysical process, but adopts a more holistic perspective in that the whole process is embraced as a unique experience for each woman. Visualised as a normative life event and essential component of women's lives, safety of mother and baby, though important, is not the only key driver. Psychosocial factors that might have a bearing on women's emotional health are also considered such as socio-cultural influences, women's wishes and feelings as well as their social and psychological needs. The social model of birth also considers women's satisfaction with their care and the environment in which birth takes place, aiming to minimise or eradicate stress factors that may give rise to unnecessary fear and anxiety (Downe et al 2008, Walsh 2007). Women and midwives travel hopefully during the intrapartum period, maintaining an optimistic view that labour and birth will be normal until proven otherwise. There is no power imbalance in such a relationship as mother and midwife are both empowered, ensuring partnership working coupled with mutual respect and trust in each other's abilities (Kirkham 2000). Therefore, the physiological process of labour and birth is nurtured and protected, and progresses without unnecessary interference, interruptions or medical interventions, and the midwife remains firmly 'with woman'. The medical model in comparison favours a technological approach and medical intervention as pregnancy, labour and birth are construed as a disease process or at least altered physiological states that have the potential to malfunction. Consequently, labour and birth are seen as a perilous journey that can only be proven as normal in retrospect (WHO 1999). This has resulted in a rather pessimistic viewpoint that over the years has created a 'just in case' policy, which attempts to justify medical interventions in normal physiological births (Mead and Kornbrot 2004). The issue of safety drives the medical model with very little regard for the psychosocial needs and feelings of the woman as care is characterised by technology and medicine (Tew 1998). Thus the woman becomes a patient – a passive recipient of care – to be controlled and managed like a machine with scant regard for her psychosocial needs (Blaaka and Schauer 2008). The experience for the woman is, therefore, very much a disembodying one as the tendency to treat her as an incubator for her baby, or a machine to be manipulated and monitored just in case her body should malfunction or go wrong is all too real.

A critical analysis of the differing models of pregnancy and childbirth as outlined by van Teijlingen (2005) identifies the different levels on which medicalisation can operate, namely: the conceptual, institutional and practitioner–mother level. Suggesting that competing and conflicting models of practice do not necessarily become a self-fulfilling prophesy by resulting in conflict in practice. Rather, van Teijlingen (2005) outlines the limitations and dichotomy that such competing models pose. He claims that a source of confusion stems from three different analytical perspectives or levels, which are summarised in Figure 6.2.

van Teijlingen (2005) states that:

Sometimes these divergent views of pregnancy and childbirth overlap, and are difficult to disentangle. As a result, students of childbirth are liable to fall into the trap of simply describing a working practice and/ or propounding its associated ideology rather than adopting an analytical approach to the issue.

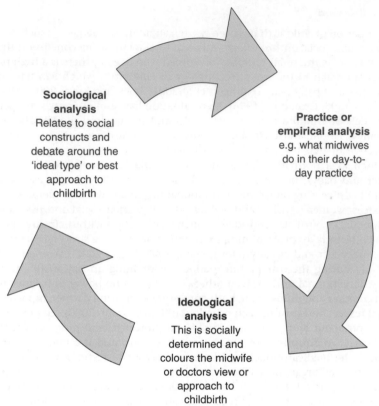

Sociological analysis
Relates to social constructs and debate around the 'ideal type' or best approach to childbirth

Practice or empirical analysis
e.g. what midwives do in their day-to-day practice

Ideological analysis
This is socially determined and colours the midwife or doctors view or approach to childbirth

Figure 6.2 A conceptual approach to the different analytical levels by which medicalisation can operate (van Teijlingen 2005)

Organisational structures: the culture of the NHS

Although the majority of women who give birth in the UK are healthy and have a 'normal' physiological labour and birth, currently there is a significant likelihood that in the majority of births occurring in NHS hospitals, women will experience some form of medical intervention during labour (NHS Information Centre 2009). This is despite influential social policies (DH 2004, 2006, 2007, WAG 2005), key recommendations from national guidelines (NICE 2007) and WHO (1999) emphasise that birth is not a medical event but a 'normal' process. In the context of normality, medical intervention does not have a place and should not be offered or recommended where labour is progressing normally. In England the government has pledged that all women will have the option of a home birth by 2009 (DH 2007), and as previously identified, to achieve this vision or 'choice guarantees' requires a seismic shift in the culture, organisation and delivery of care within the NHS. The hospital setting is still very much the dominant environment where birth takes place, and due to the shortage of midwives it is the place where the woman is least likely to experience one-to-one care or the continuous presence of a named midwife, unless the woman births in a midwife-led unit or birth centre (Hatem et al 2008). Although nationally the birth rate has increased, the rate of medical intervention has not declined significantly.

Fertility rate figures for England and Wales released by the Office of National Statistics (ONS 2008) revealed that the total number of live births increased 3% between 2006 and 2007 from 669,601 in 2006 to 690,013 in 2007, amounting to a steady increase in live births since 2001 – the highest figure since 1991, when live births reached 699,217. According to figures from the NHS Information Centre (2009) in England, the number of births occurring in NHS hospitals increased by 20,630 (3.3%) to 649, 837 in 2007–2008.

The birth rate has also increased in Scotland according to statistics released by NHS National Services Scotland (2008) and the General Registrar Office for Scotland (2009). There were 60,041 (reportedly the highest since 1995) registered live births in 2008 in Scotland compared to 55,064 live births in 2007. In England, figures from the NHS Information Centre (2009) illuminate how the pattern of birth is changing and convey a worrying trend in relation to interventions in childbirth that has a direct impact on the 'normal' birth rate as highlighted in Box 6.1.

Box 6.1 Maternity Statistics from the NHS Information Centre (2009) for England

- About 649,837 births occur in hospital settings 2007–2008 compared to 629,207 births in 2006–2007. An increase in birth rate by 3.3%.
- In 2006–2007 about 2.6% (15,900) women birthed at home an increase by 2.3% when compared to earlier years. Current figures are soon to be published by the Office of National Statistics (ONS).
- In 2007–2008, 60.3% of births were facilitated by midwives and 36.2% by doctors. That leaves approximately 3% of births unaccounted for – it is unclear whether these were births where no midwife or doctor in attendance. In 2006–2007, 62% of births were facilitated by midwives and 35% by doctors.
- There is a steady decline in 'normal' births in comparison to the 1990s when approximately 24% of births were assisted by doctors and 74% by midwives.
- In 2006–2007, 52% of births were classified as 'normal' i.e. labour was not induced, augmented, no surgical intervention/operative births or Caesarean section (LSCS), epidural or general anaesthetic. The trend is similar for 2007–2008.

The alternatives

In maternity care women's satisfaction with their care is an important determinant of health outcomes that is used by policy makers and commissioners of the service for quality assurance purposes (Goodman et al 2004). Listening to women (Sakala et al 2006) and learning from their experiences is a key part of midwifery practice. Verity's story poignantly captures the voice of many women who have exercised their choice in having a home birth.

Verity's story

In March 2008 I had a wonderful home birth with my second son, Rupert. The experience was so positive that it led to an immensely rewarding period of postnatal euphoria which in turn informed my sense of self-esteem and my mothering of my newborn child.

My approach to childbirth has always been a positive one. My mother's tales of her own three births had a profound influence on me as I was growing up. Her stories were always full of a sense of joy and wonder at the power of nature and our bodies' abilities. She had ambitions for a home birth with all three of her children. When I became pregnant myself for the first time my natural instinct was to opt for a home birth. However as my pregnancy approached 42 weeks, I agreed to be induced at my local hospital. I found the experience stressful and dis-empowering. I became very scared, very early on in the process. I felt I had to fight to be heard and found that my birth experience descended into a depressingly predictable cascade of interventions. With the help of a very supportive midwife I achieved a vaginal birth but to me the clinical induction process led to a very weak bonding with my newborn son. I carried much of the anxiety from the two day induction through to my early mothering and this anxiety combined with my feelings of detach-ment (which I link to the epidural and not having felt myself birth my child) led to me developing postnatal depression. It took me over two years to recover from this depression and left me determined to make changes in my care choices for my second pregnancy.

It was vitally important to me to have a care giver who supported my choices and who was working to support me in achieving the outcomes I desired and so I decided to work directly with an independent midwife. I carried a lot of residual anger and fear from my first birth and I felt that I needed help during the pregnancy to work through those feelings to leave me free of anxiety for the birth. I had decided not to have any ante-natal scans (I had found them emotionally uncomfortable in my first pregnancy and had come into contact with a very negative reaction when I had refused consent for markers). I also decided that I would not consider induction of labour purely based on having a post dates pregnancy and I was able to discuss these decisions with my midwife, Nicky, and was assured of her support. We built a relationship based on mutual trust and when the birth became imminent, we anticipated it together with real excitement. It was wonderful to know who would be attending my birth. It enabled me to relax about the possibility of transferring into hospital as I knew I would have someone I trusted to be my mouthpiece in that environment. I could filter information given to me by the hospital staff through her and get a balanced view of my options. It was a huge relief.

The days leading up to my labour were filled with false labour over several nights when my contractions would start at 2am and then grumble along as I slept fitfully. They would then rail off at 6am when my son woke up. I was getting really tired and grumpy but determined to wait for things to start naturally. I was really looking forward to finding out how my body would feel as it progressed through the differing intensities of contractions.

At 12 days overdue after putting my son to bed I felt as though the Braxton Hicks contractions I had been experiencing throughout the day (my midwife and I referred to them as 'surges' or 'opening sensations' to support positive visualization during the labour), seemed to be settling into more of a rhythm and my husband and I decided to wait to see if they were intensifying and becoming more frequent, before filling the birthing pool set up in our dining room. I had lit some tea lights which I had dotted around the room in preparation, turned off the main light and bounced on my ball watching some TV. We kept looking at each other and grinning shyly wondering if this was truly it. We were so excited about what was about to happen. I had no nerves or fear, I was so joyous that I was starting labour as nature intended, slowly and in the comfort of my own nest.

A short while later I called my midwife to tell her I thought things might be getting started. Not long after this call I had a contraction which left me anxious and reminded me of the fear I had felt in the hospital. I knew I wanted Nicky with me as soon as possible to bring her calming presence to the room. At 1am, she arrived and quietly slipped in, hiding the canisters of gas and air behind a chair. At the same time as calling my midwife I called my mum who came round and attempted to sleep upstairs to be available to whisk my son away when he woke in the morning as we had arranged. I had no concerns about him witnessing my labour and birth but felt I would like to be able to give my undivided attention to this amazing event and that with him present I wouldn't be able to do this. Mum was also very sensitive to my needs and tip toed in without a word during a contraction and went straight upstairs. I had started earlier in the evening using some vocalization to see if it helped with the sensations during a surge but quickly abandoned that when I realized that concentrating on slow, deep breathing took me to another place and kept my focus away from my womb and the feeling of the muscles working to open my cervix. I felt so drugged up on my own hormones and so deeply focused on my self-hypnosis that I really had to take a minute to 'come round' after each contraction. Sitting down on my ball ensured my contractions continued to strengthen and standing up lessened their effectiveness so when I needed a break I would stand but mainly I enjoyed driving them on by staying seated. Nicky was a very quiet presence and my husband was sleeping on the sofa for a couple of these hours as I felt perfectly self-contained and was happy simply to have his presence in the room. Nicky simply murmured a few words of gentle, positive encouragement when she could see that I was struggling to focus. It was on these rare occasions as the contractions changed in intensity level that I would experience the sensations as what I would call sharp pain. I got into the pool for a while and enjoyed a relaxing break as my contractions slowed to a more manageable level but knew that I would need to get out to get things moving along again so did so. I was thrilled to be able to reattach the tens machine I had been using as this was a really useful diversionary tool, shifting my focus away from the centre of the surge to the sensation on my back.

At dawn my son woke up and he and mum walked through the room to leave for the day. It was lovely to explain to him that I was having the baby and that we were all very excited and I would see him soon. We had a kiss and he trotted off happily. Shortly after this I dropped to my knees on the sitting room floor and started swaying my hips in a yoga move I had learnt. I was starting to say that I needed something more to help with the feelings, water or gas and air. We opted for water first and I resumed my floating position.

Nicky went for a short power nap during which I was quietly sick into a bowl. I was delighted to be sick as I knew this meant I was opening up really well and my body was preparing itself for the birth. All my thoughts were so positive and I keep expressing my excitement that all this was happening and how lucky I and my baby were to be having this experience together. It was so different to this stage in my previous labour.

It wasn't long before I decided the time really had come for the gas and air and Nicky asked if she could do an internal examination (the first and only of her visit) to establish where I was in my labour. I knew I was well progressed and was happy for this examination to go ahead. She told us I was 7–8 centimetres and it was a glistening moment of joy in the whole experience. Jim and I had a little laugh, clap and general celebration as we knew then that we had done it! We were having our home birth and I had gone through the hardest, longest part. It was just a short distance to travel to the actual arrival of our new child. My thoughts became much more lucid as my contractions got closer together and the spaces between them shortened. Although I felt as though I had all the time in the world between contractions to gather my strength – it was a very serene part of the labour. My transition from opening to pushing came over several longer contractions when I started to sing long loud notes, and then my body was pushing. It was all happening so fast at one point I felt as though the expulsive contractions wouldn't end so I flipped over onto my back (easy to do in the water), and felt more able to focus my energies. It was the most wonderful sensation feeling my baby's head move down my birth canal. I was unable to put my hand down to protect my perineum as Jim was asking me to, so after a quick feel to assure myself how far out the head was, I gave an almighty push and Jim caught our baby's head and then body as he was born all in one push. It was such a simple process. I sat and wondered at my baby and fell head over heels in love, then after a short while stood to birth the placenta before moving into the sitting room to lie on the sofa and breast feed.

Gabriel came home a couple of hours later and met his new brother as we all lay in bed tired but euphoric. The birth was an immensely important achievement in my life and has been a very healing experience. I was struck by how undramatic having a child at home is – with the right care around you it can be such a gentle and life affirming event.

Verity could afford an independent midwife, but not all women are in a financial position to exercise this choice. NHS maternity care in the UK is free, and arguably, independent midwifery should be a viable option for women if healthcare providers could commission this service. Care within the NHS would then allow for happy stories and good outcomes like Verity's.

Women who do not wish to birth at home or in a hospital consultant-led unit, a midwife-led unit or a birth centre provides the ideal alternative and a half-way house. They offer a family centred environment that on evaluation reveals psychological benefits for women (Downe 2008, Hatem et al 2008, Hodnett et al 2007, Walsh 2006, Kirkham 2003) as outlined in Box 6.2. Birth centres and midwife-led units are terms used interchangeably and synonymously. They can be 'stand alone' or integrated into larger maternity units as a separate space from the consultant-led labour suite, which is staffed and managed by highly skilled midwives. This alternative environment offers a relaxed, comfortable, ambient, low technology, friendly and welcoming space, where care is individualised and geared towards meeting the needs of women and their family. Organisational structures supporting midwifery-led care should ensure that there is scope for early labour assessment in women's home or triage facilities, where the woman can make informed decisions regarding the birth environment of her choosing (Spiby and Renfrew 2008, Cheyne et al 2007, Lauzon and Hodnett 2001).

Box 6.2 Psychological benefits of midwife-led units/birth centres

- Increased sense of control, promotes psychophysical harmony as there are less confounding variables that can result in fear, stress and anxiety
- More likelihood of woman experiencing 1:1 care from a midwife diminishing the need for the woman to use pharmacological means of analgesia
- Less likelihood of interventions such as lower segment caesarean section, instrumental birth, induction, augmentation and episiotomy
- Midwives adopt an unhurried approach and embrace the philosophy of a woman-centred approach to care to ensure that women are firmly in the driving seat
- Women more likely to express satisfaction with their birth experience and succeed at breastfeeding

Perception of pain: psychological factors

Pain is not just a sensory experience that results from stimulation of specific nerve receptors: it is a complex biophysical phenomenon that is also mediated by emotions, cognitive processes and other psychosocial factors such as environment. Whether the environment is too hot or too cold, distracting or over-stimulating to the senses, a source of tension or a haven of calm and relaxation will all impact on the woman's perception of pain. The DH (2004) states that the birth environment should aim to promote normality and take account of women's choice and wishes, which is echoed in the results of a survey published by the National Childbirth Trust (NCT) (Newburn and Singh 2003). The four key areas of importance when considering a woman's perception of pain are:

1. Empathy
2. Support
3. Partnership
4. Environment that the labouring woman rates as quiet, relaxed and comfortable.

As outlined in Chapter 5, empathetic listening and attending tend to come in the guise of skilled help by midwives who are facilitative in their approach rather than obstructive or hinder normal progress during labour. Support provided by birth companions that the woman chooses will have a beneficial effect by reducing the woman's need for pharmacological analgesia (Hodnett et al 2007). This is the only intervention during labour that seems to result in a positive outcome for mothers and babies (Green et al 1998). Partnership, providing woman-centred care, respects the autonomy of the woman, supports and involves her in decision-making (VandeVusse 1999), and at the same time acknowledges tacit ways of knowing such as the woman's ability to use her intuitive knowledge in birthing her baby (Newburn and Singh 2003). A birth environment that is quiet, relaxed and comfortable is more likely to help ameliorate stress factors and promote psychophysical harmony, enabling important hormones such as oxytocin, endorphins and encephalin to flow freely. Simkin et al (2001) identify three characteristics that assist women to cope well with the stresses and pain of labour, which is referred to as the three Rs: relaxation, rhythm and ritual.

Hormones of love

The work of Dick-Read (2004) attests to hormonal influences on the progress of labour. He likens the labouring woman to other mammals who share the basic psychological need to feel safe, protected and secure in order that the process of labour and birth can progress normally. Fear he argues is the most protective of all emotions and a powerful contributory cause of pain. From a cultural perspective the fear of labour and childbirth (**tokophobia**) is deeply engrained in the psyche of many Western women. They no longer observe other women within their households giving birth, but experience it by television and other popular media. This results in childbirth being feared and seen as highly dangerous and a very painful experience. Equally, hospitalisation of birth has created a medicalised view of the process with very little understanding of the dimension and purpose of uterine contractions. Hence many women see childbirth as something to be feared and endured. Pain in childbirth is a misconception that has no place in normal physiological labour, Dick-Read (2004) reports. Pain he asserts is a sympathetic response via the nervous system – the direct result of fear that creates tension leading to what he terms the 'fear-tension-pain syndrome as outlined in Figure 6.3.

Dick-Read's (2004) theory gave birth to the notion of antenatal education and preparation classes to equip women with the understanding of how their mental abilities can be used in a positive way to influence the course of labour and result in natural childbirth. In many ways this equates to **psychoprophylaxis** or the ubiquitously stated axiom, 'mind over matter'. Fear releases stress hormones: cortisol and catecholamine (noradrenaline and adrenaline) which cause marked changes in the cardiovascular system due to their effect of vasoconstriction. Psychologically, this impacts on the labouring woman and fetus in a number of ways, the corollary of which is outlined in Box 6.3.

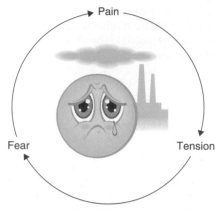

Figure 6.3 The Cyclical Dimension of Pain (Dick-Read 2004)

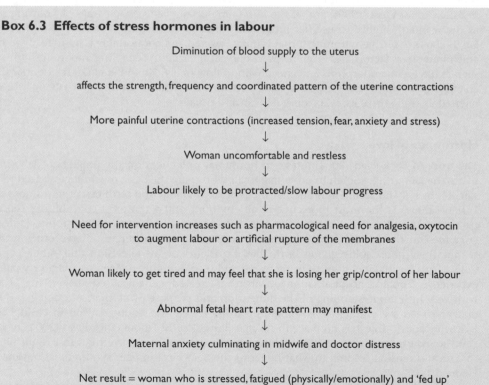

Box 6.3 Effects of stress hormones in labour

Diminution of blood supply to the uterus
↓
affects the strength, frequency and coordinated pattern of the uterine contractions
↓
More painful uterine contractions (increased tension, fear, anxiety and stress)
↓
Woman uncomfortable and restless
↓
Labour likely to be protracted/slow labour progress
↓
Need for intervention increases such as pharmacological need for analgesia, oxytocin to augment labour or artificial rupture of the membranes
↓
Woman likely to get tired and may feel that she is losing her grip/control of her labour
↓
Abnormal fetal heart rate pattern may manifest
↓
Maternal anxiety culminating in midwife and doctor distress
↓
Net result = woman who is stressed, fatigued (physically/emotionally) and 'fed up'

Odent (1999) builds on the foundations of the hormonal influences of labour, especially the role of oxytocin coining it as the 'love hormone'. He provides scientific explanations for the role of oxytocin and its complex interactions in human behaviour during some of the most intimate moments such as coitus, conception, labour (all stages) and birth as well as lactation. Intimacy needs privacy, reports Odent (1999), without it oxytocin will be inhibited. Midwives, therefore, must ensure that the birth environment enables the dynamics of the neuro-hormonal reflex to take place and assist women in developing a clear understanding of the inter-relationship between pregnancy events and childbirth. This means providing information on the ebb and flow of uterine contractions, that they are not a constant but the woman will experience reprieve between each energy surge, allowing her to gather her inner strength and focus on the power of her body. To do this, women need specific tools to create a road map to help themselves navigate the physiological processes involved in labour and birth (Simkin et al 2001).

Factors influencing perception of pain

A woman's experience of pain will be influenced not only by the intensity of the sensory stimuli but on the perception, thought and emotions and generally how the experience is dealt with cognitively. Modulators of pain or coping strategies also play an important role, and there are several ways in which the labouring woman can engage or utilise her power or sense of self-efficacy to master pain sensations. These include a sense of control and employment of cognitive techniques such as distraction, relaxation or visualisation.

Conclusion

Although many factors can influence a woman's experience of labour and birth, the physical environment in which birth takes place can have a profound impact on her psychological and emotional wellbeing. This may result from the amount of choice and control she has over decision-making to the degree of tension, fear and anxiety she experiences (Hodnett et al 2005). In their own environment women often have the undivided attention of a skilled midwife, the self-belief and the powerful effects of oxytocin to ensure progress in labour. Yet, less than 3% of women with uncomplicated pregnancies have a home birth in the UK. Verity's story is the exception rather than the rule. This is despite the growing evidence to dispel the myth that hospital is the safest environment for babies to be born (de Jonge et al 2009, Johnson and Daviss 2005). Birth in hospital can be an alienating experience for women due to routine procedures, lack of privacy and more likelihood of women being left alone for long periods (HCC 2008); thus usurping their coping abilities and increasing the demand for pharmacological analgesia (Hodnett et al 2007). Medical intervention is also more likely as well as the birth becoming a technical performance rather than a spontaneous human birth. In an effort to keep birth 'normal' for those women who do not wish to remain at home, birth centres and midwife-led units offer a real alternative from the hustle and bustle and impersonal nature of more traditional maternity units (Downe et al 2008, Hatem et al 2008, Walsh 2007, Kirkham 2003).

Summary of key points

- There is no evidence to suggest that women presenting with uncomplicated pregnancies should not have a choice of birth environment (NICE 2007, WAG 2005, DH 2004).

- In the UK the evidence to support the claim that a planned home birth is just as safe as birth in the hospital setting is conflicting and unreliable (Gyte et al 2009, Mori et al 2008), although there are some encouraging studies from other countries (de Jonge et al 2009).

- Control and choice are important to women's experience of childbirth and an integral part of their psychological needs and emotional wellbeing (Hatem et al 2008, Green et al 1998).

- Home births or a home-like environment such as birth centres or midwifery-led units are associated with greater maternal satisfaction with care, reduced need for pharmacological analgesia, reduced medical interventions such as augmentation of labour and instrumental births as women are more likely to feel in control and experience one-to-one care (Hatem et al 2008, Hodnett et al 2005, 2007, Kirkham 2003, Simkin and O'Hara 2002).

- There should be scope for early labour assessment in women's homes or triage facilities where the woman can make informed decisions regarding the best place for her to have her baby (Spiby and Renfrew 2008, Cheyne et al 2007, Lauzon and Hodnett 2001).

- Births in hospitals that are medically dominated are more likely to result in a disempowering experience for women due to hospital routines, medicalisation, lack of privacy and less likelihood of the woman receiving continuous support from a named midwife (HCC 2008, Redshaw et al 2007).

References

Blaaka, G. and Schauer, T. (2008) Doing midwifery between different belief systems. *Midwifery*, 24(3): 344–52.

Campbell, R. and Macfarlane, A. (1994) *Where to be Born: the debate and the evidence*, 2nd edn. Oxford: NPEU.

Chamberlain, G., Wraight, A. and Crowley, P. (1997) *Homebirths*. Carnford: Pergamon.

Cheyne, H., Terry, R., Niven, C., Dowding, D., Hundley, V. and McNamee, P. (2007) 'Should I come in now?': a study of women's early labour experiences. *British Journal of Midwifery*, 15(10): 604–9.

Crompton, J. (1996) Post-traumatic stress disorder and childbirth: 2. *British Journal of Midwifery*, 4(7): 354–73.

de Jonge, A., van der Goes, B.Y. 2nd, Ravelli, A.C.J. (2009) Perinatal mortality and morbidity in a nationwide cohort of 529 688 low-risk planned home and hospital births. *British Journal of Obstetrics and Gynaecology*, 116: 1–8.

Department of Health (2007) *Maternity Matters: Access and continuity of care in a safe service*. London: DH.

Department of Health (2006) *Our Health, our Care, our Say*. London: DH.

Department of Health (2004) *National Service Framework for Children, Young People and Maternity Service* (Standard 11). London: DH.

Dick-Read, G. (2004) *Childbirth without Fear: the principles and practice of natural childbirth*. London: Pinter and Martin.

Downe, S. (ed.) (2008) *Normal Childbirth: evidence and debate*, 2nd edn. Edinburgh: Churchill Livingstone.

Downe, S., Walsh, D. and Gyte, G.T. (2008) Is maternity care evidence based or interpretation driven? Place of birth as an exemplar. *Midwifery*, 24(3): 247–9.

General Registrar Office for Scotland (2009) News release: Births increase for the sixth consecutive year. http://www.gro-scotland.gov.uk.

Goodman, P., Mackey, M.C. and Tavakoli, A.S. (2004) Factors related to childbirth satisfaction. *Journal of Advanced Nursing*, 46(2): 212–19.

Green, J.M., Coupland, V.A. and Kitzinger, J.V. (1998) *Great Expectations: a prospective study of women's expectations and experiences of childbirth*, 2nd edn. Hale: Books for Midwives Press.

Gyte, G., Dodwell, M., Newburn, C., Sandall, J., Macfarlane, A. and Bewley, S. (2009) Estimating intrapartum-related perinatal mortality rates for booked homebirths: when the 'best' available data are not good enough. *British Journal of Obstetrics and Gynaecology*, 116: 933–42.

Hatem, M., Sandall, J., Devane, D., Soltani, H. and Gates, S. (2008) Midwife-led versus other models of care for childbearing women. *Cochrane Database of Systematic Reviews*. Art No: CD004667. DOI: 10.10021/14651858.

Healthcare Commission (2008) *Towards Better Births: a review of maternity services in England*. http://www.cqc.org.uk, accessed 12 April 2009.

Hodnett, E.D., Gates, S., Hofmeyr, G.J. and Sakala, C. (2007) Continuous support for women during childbirth (Review). *Cochrane Database of Systematic Reviews*, Issue 3. Art No: CD003766.DOI:10.1002/14651858.

Hodnett, E.D., Downe, S., Edwards, N. and Walsh, D. (2005) Home-like versus conventional institutional settings for birth (Review). *Cochrane Database of Systematic Reviews*, Issue 1. Art No: CD000012. DOI: 10.1002/14651858D.

Hunter, B. (2009) The emotional context of midwifery. In: D. Fraser, M.A. Cooper (eds) *Myles Textbook for Midwives*, 15th edn. London: Churchill Livingstone, pp 11–19.

Hunter, B. (2006) The importance of reciprocity in relationships between community based midwives and mothers. *Midwifery*, 22(4): 308–22.

Janssen, P.A., Saxell, L., Page, L.A., Klein, M.C., Liston, R.M. and Lee, S.K. (2009) Outcomes of planned home birth with registered midwife vs planned hospital birth with midwife or physician. *Canadian Medical Association Journal*, DOI 10.1503/cmaj.081869.

Johnson, K.G. and Daviss, B.A. (2005) Outcomes of planned home births with certified professional midwives: large prospective study in North America. *British Medical Journal*, 330: 1416–22.

Kirkham, M. (ed.) (2003) *Birth Centres: a social model for maternity care*. Oxford: Books for Midwives Press.

Kirkham, M. (2000) How can we relate? In: M. Kirkham (ed.) *The Midwife–Woman Relationship*. Basingstoke: Palgrave Macmillan, pp 227–50.

Kirkham, M. (1999) The culture of midwifery in the National Health Service in England. *Journal of Advanced Nursing*, 30: 732–9.

Lauzon, L. and Hodnett, E.D. (2001) Labour assessment programs to delay admission to labour wards. *Cochrane Database of Systematic Reviews*, Issue 3. Art No: CD000936 DOI:10.1002/14651858.

Mead, M.M.P. and Kornbrot, D. (2004) The influence of maternity units intrapartum intervention rates and midwives risk perception for women suitable for midwifery-led care. *Midwifery*, 20(1): 61–71.

Mori, R., Dougherty, M. and Whittle, M. (2008) An estimation of intrapartum-related perinatal mortality rates for booked home births in England and Wales between 1994 and 2003. *British Journal of Obstetrics and Gynaecology*, 115: 554–9.

National Institute for Health and Clinical Excellence (2007) *Intrapartum Care: care of healthy women and their babies during childbirth*. CG55: London: NICE.

National Perinatal Epidemiology Unit (2008) *The Birthplace in England Research Programme (Birthplace)*. http://www.npeu.ox.ac.uk, accessed 22 April 2009.

Newburn, M. and Singh, D. (2003) *Creating a Better Birth Environment: women's' views about the design and facilities in maternity units*. A national survey for the NCT. London: National Childbirth Trust.

NHS Information Centre (2009) *NHS Maternity Statistics, England: 2007–2008*. http://www.ic.nhs.uk, accessed 5 May 2009.

NHS National Services Scotland (2008) *Births and Babies*. http://www.isdscotland.org, accessed 19 April 2009.

Odent, M. (1999) *The Scientification of Love*, revised edition. London: Free Association Press.

Office of National Statistics (2008) News release: Fertility rate highest for 34 years. http://www.statistics.gov.uk, accessed 20 April 2009.

Olsen, O. and Jewell, D. (1998) Home versus hospital birth. *Cochrane Database of Systematic Reviews*, Issue 3. Art No: CD000352. DOI: 10.1002/14651858.

Page, L. (2006) An ideal birth environment? The right facilities and support for women. *British Journal of Midwifery*, 4(1): 46.

Redshaw, M., Rowe, R., Hockley, C. and Brocklehurst, P. (2007) *Recorded Delivery: a national survey of women's experience of maternity care 2006*. Oxford: NPEU.

Royal College of Midwives (2008) *Birth Environment: evidence based guidelines for midwifery led care in labour*, 4th edn. http://www.rcm.org.uk, accessed 20 April 2009.

Sakala, C., Declercq, E.R. and Corry, M.P. (2006) Listening to mothers. The first national survey of women's childbearing experiences. *Journal of Obstetrics, Gynecology and Neonatal Nursing*, 31(6): 633–4.

Sandin-Bojö, A.K. and Kvist, L.J. (2008) Care in labor: a Swedish survey using the Bologna Score. *Birth*, 35(4): 321–8.

Savage, W. (2007) *Birth and Power: a savage enquiry revisited*. London: Middlesex Press.

Simkin, P. and O'Hara, M. (2002) Non-pharmacological relief of pain during labour: systematic review of five methods. *American Journal of Obstetrics and Gynecology*, 186: S131–S159.

Simkin, P., Whaley, J. and Kipper, A. (2001) *Pregnancy, Childbirth and the Newborn: the complete guide*. New York: Meadowbrook.

Spiby, H. and Renfrew, E.G. (2008) Achieving the best care in early labour. *BUJ*, 337:a1165 online journal. www.bmj.com/cgi/content/full/337/aug28_1/a1021, accessed 20 April 2009.

Stapleton, H., Kirkham, M., Thomas, G. and Curtis, P. (2002) Midwives in the middle: balance and vulnerability. *British Journal of Midwifery*, 10(10): 607–11.

Steer, P. (2008) How safe is home birth? Editor's choice. *British Journal of Obstetrics and Gynaecology*, 115: i–ii.

Stockhill, C. (2007) Trust the experts? A commentary on choice and control in childbirth. *Feminism and Psychology*, 17(4): 571–7.

Tew, M. (1998) Safer childbirth? *A Critical History of Maternity Care*, 3rd edn. London: Chapman Hall.

Tracy, S. and Tracy, M. (2003) Costing the cascade: estimating the cost of increased obstetric intervention in childbirth using population data. *British Journal of Obstetrics and Gynaecology*, 110: 717–24.

VandeVusse (1999) Decision making in analyses of women's birth stories. *Birth*, 26(1): 43–5.

van Teijlingen, E. (2005) A critical analysis of the medical model as used in the study of pregnancy and childbirth. *Sociological Research Online*, 10(2). http://www.socresonline.org.uk/10/2/teijlingen.html accessed, 20 April 2009.

van Teijlingen, E., Lowis, G., McCaffery, P. and Porter, M. (eds) (2004) *Midwifery and the Medicalization of Childbirth: comparative perspectives*, 1st edn. New York: Nova Science.

Walsh, D. (2007) *Evidence-based Care for Normal Labour and Birth: a guide for midwives*. London: Routledge.

Walsh, D. (2006) *Improving Maternity Service: small is beautiful – lessons from a birth centre*. London: Radcliffe.

Walsh, D. and Downe, S. (2008) Uncertainty around home birth transfers. *British Journal of Obstetrics and Gynaecology*, 115: 1184.

Welsh Assembly Government (2005) *National Service Framework for Children, Young People and Maternity Services – core actions for delivery by the end of March 2006*. http://www.wales.nhs.uk, accessed 19 April 2009.

Werkmeister, G., Jokinem, M., Mahmood, T. and Newburn, M. (2008) Making normal labour-birth a reality – developing a multidisciplinary consensus. *Midwifery*, 24(3): 256–9.

World Health Organization (1999) *Care in Normal Birth: a practical guide*. Geneva: WHO. http://www.who.int, accessed 10 April 2009.

Young, G., Hey, E., Macfarlane, A. et al (2000) Choosing between home and hospital birth. *British Medical Journal*, 320: 798–9.

Annotated further reading

Fahy, K., Fourer, M. and Hastie, C. (2008) *Birth Territory and Midwifery Guardianship: theory for practice, education and research*. Hale: Books for Midwives.

This text explores the salient elements of an ideal birth environment and offers some useful tips for practice.

Hunter, B. and Deery, R. (eds) (2009) *Emotions in Midwifery and Reproduction*. Basingstoke: Macmillan.

This edited text explores why emotion in midwifery and health care is important, highlighting the reciprocity of the caring relationship, i.e. 'emotion work' applies to carer and the cared for.

Welsh Assembly Government (2003) *All Wales Clinical Pathway for Normal Labour*. http://www.wales.nhs.uk/normallabour, accessed 19 April 2009.

Provides a useful benchmark for helping women to achieve normal birth.

Useful websites

www.nice.org.uk
www.who.int
www.rcm.org.uk
http://www.wales.nhs.uk
http://www.isdscotland.org
http://www.ic.nhs.uk

7 The psychology of stress, anxiety and coping

Chapter contents

Introduction

Chapter aims

Psychology of the self: self-knowledge

Defending the self from stresses and inconsistencies

The relationship between stress and coping

Coping strategies and midwifery practice

The related states of fear, anxiety, stress and emotion

Self-efficacy and coping

Control and coping

Fear, anxiety and birthing, not a winning combination

Conclusion

Summary of key points

References

Annotated further reading

Website

Introduction

Psychological stress and anxiety are behaviour states that are generally regarded as relatively normal events in childbearing, based on the notion that they are common features seen in pregnancy, childbirth and the postnatal period. This does not mean however that they are harmless as they can dramatically reduce the enjoyment and quality of a woman's childbirth experience, which is vital both to her own wellbeing and to her future relationship with her partner and child. The physiological response to a threat is via the neocortex and the limbic system, which triggers the hypothalamus and pituitary gland. The influence of cognitive appraisal of a threat on adrenaline and cortisol production renders the person's response, unique to them. Being aroused or debilitated by different degrees of stress, anxiety and/or fear is part of everyday living. Usual ways of communicating may be changed by a process of cognitive distraction as the person will sample a range of coping strategies that may enable them to deal with a simple hassle or a major life event. Coping is linked to how each person, from birth has constructed their self-concept. Self-esteem is seen as a vital component of wellbeing and will fluctuate as people assess their daily challenges and the effectiveness of their coping skills to deal with them. Perceptions of personal control and self-efficacy will contribute to this process. Keeping stress and anxiety to a minimum is a vital part of midwifery care. Stressed midwives and their obstetric team colleagues can stress parents. Added to this there is a growing body of evidence that maternal stress causes fetal stress, which may affect neurodevelopment in the baby. It is known that maternal stress will slow or stop labour and deprive the fetus of oxygen. This chapter will examine these concepts. Where the text refers to people, this means the men and women that are in receipt of care and those who are providing it in multi-agency teams and networks (DH 2008).

Chapter aims

- To explore in detail the need for each person to create and maintain a consistent sense of self

- To highlight that stress, anxiety and fear are physiological responses to cognitive appraisals that are mediated via the neocortex, limbic and autonomic nervous systems

- To suggest that stress, anxiety and fear are learned from an early age, which includes fetal life and such experiences can have a detrimental effect on neurobiological development

- To discuss how people use coping strategies to manage their threat situation

- To explore the relationship between one's perception of self-efficacy and control

- To reaffirm that stress, anxiety and fear adversely affect cognitive function, especially communications with others, which may become strained and/or stilted

---

Psychology of the self: self-knowledge

Self-knowledge is crucial in regulating and directing a person's thoughts, feelings, and behaviour in order to seek out situations that match their capabilities. Such pursuits can result in pride and joy or serve to evoke fear, even anger. Self-knowledge is constructed rather than known and is sometimes difficult for the person to understand, hence this is why some people seek help in order for them to understand how they have constructed aspects of themselves (British Association for Counselling and Psychotherapy 2009). Self-knowledge has two components: the self-concept which represents *what* a person comes to know about herself and self-esteem, *how* she feels about herself.

How the self-concept is constructed

According to Goffman (1990) people create their own behaviour from what they have observed in others. They also use thoughts and feelings and other people's reactions to form opinions about themselves. According to the *looking glass self* other people's reactions serve as a mirror to reflect a person's image, so that the person themselves can see it. If a midwife is told that she is good at student mentoring, she will tend to behave in keeping with their portrayed image of that role. However this only applies to people who are uncertain about their actual self-concept and the process is similar to the *self-fulfilling prophecy* because it is the influence of other people that is creating the change. Multiple motives lead people to compare themselves to others. These include the need for accurate self-evaluations and desires for empathy and connectedness; for inspiration from others or for positive feelings about themselves from making comparisons to others who they consider are worse off than themselves. Such influences are conceived by whom a person chooses for comparison and also what makes the person unique or distinctive from the rest. Bem (1967) argues in his Self Perception theory that people learn about themselves by observing their own behaviours in the situation in which it occurs and then infer their attitudes and values from it. People come to realise that others see them as less variable and more consistent than the ways they see themselves because a person has a greater quantity and variety of information about themselves than about others.

The self-schema

There is a tendency to attribute one's own behaviour to situational causes while seeing others act in accordance to their inner characteristics. This enables a person to interpret one's inconsistent behaviour as a result of inconsistent circumstances, not of an inconsistent self. However, in time people come to realise that they are multiple selves in the way they engage in different roles, groups and relationships and how they think, feel and act in each one (Smith 1999). So in order to construct a coherent self-concept, people limit their information accessibility to one role and ignore aspects of their other roles. Thus they construct a unified and enduring sense of self by noting a few core attributes that they believe characterises them uniquely amongst people and consistently across situations. Simon and Trötschel (2008) describe the self-schema as a cognitive generalisation about the self, derived from past social experiences that organise and guide the processing of self-related information. Once a particular characteristic is incorporated into the self-schema (I am a hard worker; I am a compassionate person), when noticed it is processed very effectively and any inconsistencies are quickly rejected, so increasing the person's sense of consistency. Bierhoff (2008) argues that there are recognised cultural differences in the self-concept, indeed members of Western independent cultures stress that self-schema traits generally describe them across situations, whilst those in interdependent cultures, emphasise their roles and relationships with others (also see Chapter 5).

Constructing self-esteem

Self-esteem is the positive or negative evaluation of the self or how one feels about oneself. It tells the person how they are doing in constructing a positive valued self that functions well, attains rewards and fosters relationships with others. People gravitate to life choices that enable them to flourish because this is more likely to result in high self-esteem, an important resource that protects the person against stress and threats to the self. The self-concept once formed is relatively difficult to change. Once particular domains of the self are established, inconsistent feedback is avoided, distrusted or resisted, even if it is flattering. This function of the self is important in creating a sense of a stable personal identity making the person subjectively the same person each day. People with an unstable or fluctuating self-concept tend to have low self-esteem which illustrates the value of having a secure and certain sense of self.

The self and emotions

Emotions mark the most meaningful moments in an individual's life and feelings like pride, joy, anxiety, fear or anger signal that something *important* to the self is happening. The intrusive nature of emotions forces the person to pay attention to significant events. Emotions are complex and involve the entire self, body and mind, action and thought. The limbic system, known as the emotional brain, controls emotional responses to external stimuli (see Box 7.2 and Figure 7.1). Consider in Case vignette 7.1 how certain forms of information can trigger cognitive attention.

Case vignette 7.1

Rebecca and Russell were preparing to take home their two-day-old baby Beth. Their named midwife performed the examination of the newborn screening assessment and in handing Beth back to her mother, informed the parents that Beth had a heart murmur. Both parents initially responded with stunned silence (see Box 7.1). The news was followed up with further information that heart murmurs are a common finding at this time and a second opinion would be immediately sought. The midwife spoke in an unhurried confident way, in soft tones and invited them both to ask any questions. When they were composed enough to be left, the midwife rang the neonatal registrar and asked her to attend. Beth was re-examined, the murmur was confirmed and Rebecca was asked to stay in hospital so that Beth could be further assessed. The following morning, the same registrar examined Beth to find that the murmur was no longer detectable. The parents decided to take Beth home that morning.

Box 7.1 Emotional and bio-physiological responses which may be seen when a person is in receipt of significant news/information

Racing heart rate

Pounding head, feeling faint

Feeling sick

Feeling anger

Sweating

Inability to think, feeling confused, disorientated

Disbelief

Overwhelming panic

Wanting to scream

Guilt

Stunned silence

Smith and Mackie (2007) assert that different cognitive appraisals of the same situation can produce different emotions. They believe there are two types of appraisals:

1. Whether the event is seen as positive or negative. An event that is perceived as supportive to the self-concept may generate feelings of hope or gratitude whereas an unsupportive appraisal may lead to feelings of threat, frustration, fear, anger or disgust.
2. Who or what causes or controls the event. If there is someone to blame, one may ask: is the fault mine or is it someone else's responsibility?

The emotions one feels and actions subsequently taken will be different depending on the answers to these two questions. Many factors influence the way a person will appraise an event and will include the context, their accessible thoughts and transient moods. Other people's reactions play a part in how a person responds too. The labels that are applied to the person's inner feelings are often based on salient cues, conspicuous features, people or events that may or may not correspond to the true cause of the emotion.

These are factors that may have influenced how Rebecca and Russell cognitively appraised their situation:

- the supportive attitude and confident behaviour of the midwife
- the way the news was imparted with clear, precise information, soft tone of voice, good timing
- no suggestion that the news was bad or urgent. News is neutral and this principle was upheld so that the parents were free to appraise it, as they perceived it

- there was appropriate follow-up information and a practical plan of action with no long delays
- the parents responded to the request for Rebecca to stay in hospital as reasonable
- the parents were able to decide when they wished to go home which confirmed their sense of control and confidence in the managed interventions and outcome of the situation
- at no time was blame apportioned to any person.

Sometimes a salient object may not be the real cause of an emotion. For example a midwife may experience feelings of anger toward an annoying colleague, but it could be related to the way she was treated earlier in the day. Strong emotions of any sort, positive or negative, can create intense arousal that limit a person's ability to pay attention to other events. Cognitive appraisals of an event, physical feelings from the body (raised heart beat) and emotionally driven behaviour are frequently activated together (Woolsey et al 2008). As a result they can become associated so that any one aspect can engage all the rest (see Case vignette 7.2).

Box 7.2 The limbic system – the emotional brain

The limbic system is a collection of nuclei and tracts that border the thalamus and comprises of the amygdala, mammillary body, hippocampus and fornix. Added to this is the olfactory bulb, the septum, cortex of the cingulated gyrus and the hypothalamus (see Figure 7.1). The limbic system is involved in the regulation of motivated behaviours in comprehending the emotional significance of situations and events (Nolte 2007). According to Crossman and Neary (2005) information from the outside world is collected through visual, auditory and touch pathways via the thalamus with the exception of the olfactory system, which is the only major sensory pathway that reaches the cerebral cortex without passing through the thalamus (Pinel 2006). The olfactory cortex and hippocampal cortex make up 10% of the total cerebral cortex and are often referred to as the primitive or paleocortex (old cortex) because of their early evolutionary origins. About 90% of the cerebral cortex is called the neocortex (new cortex).

Entry of information to the limbic system is either directly to the amygdala (pronounced a-MIG-dah-lah) or indirectly to the hippocampus which processes experience into memories and is involved in the recall of spacial locations. The amygdala integrates information from the senses and visceral sensations from the body with past experience and is specifically involved in perceiving facial expressions of emotion particularly of fear or negative emotions and the emotional tone of the voice, which is called prosody. When the amygdala receives input from all sensory systems, it learns the emotionally significant signals and retains them. A pathway from the amygdala to the peri-aqueductal grey area of the midbrain (an endorphin sensitive circuit that blocks pain) and to the lateral hypothalamus, elicit appropriate sympathetic responses.

Over time, conditioning stimuli that enter the amygdala trigger pathways that ultimately result in a fear response. Environments or contexts, in which fear-inducing stimuli are encountered, can themselves come to elicit fear, a process called contextual fear conditioning. The hospital context is a common example of this phenomenon.

The right hemisphere is dominant in the perception of emotion for both facial expression and tone. Facial expressions develop sooner and are of greater magnitude on the left side of the face, which is controlled by the right hemisphere (Pinel 2006). The limbic system then sends motor responses to the basal ganglion for refinement, before sending them to the body via the hypothalamus and brain stem.

From a bio-psychological perspective, the power of odours, past experiences, tone of voice and facial expressions cannot be over-emphasised in the way people respond to certain stimuli. Midwives will not know what stimuli may trigger which woman in what way and can be applied to the midwife herself. Working with emotionally stressed and anxious women can be highly contagious. An anxious midwife can have a deleterious effect upon a coping woman.

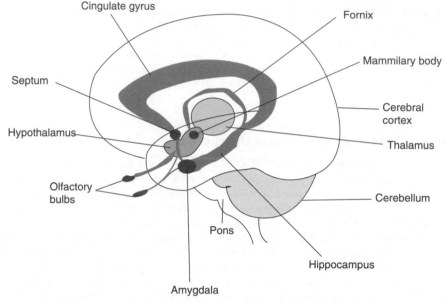

Figure 7.1 To show the limbic system structures and their relationships to other cerebral landmarks

Case vignette 7.2

Lisa and John were having their second baby and had come to the hospital for an anomaly scan at 20 weeks gestation. Their first baby had been found dead at this examination so it was an anxious time for them. When they were called into the scan room, Lisa became distressed and tearful. She did not wish to be scanned by her assigned ultrasonographer or to be in the room with her. She later described to the midwife that her memories of the first pregnancy scan had 'came flooding back to her' and she had re-lived the emotions of that situation and was now experiencing extreme fear of losing this baby. The ultrasonographer was relatively familiar with this reaction and quickly made alternative arrangements for Lisa to be examined by a colleague. Afterwards when Lisa had seen and heard her live baby on scan, she was able to speak to the ultrasonographer and express her feelings. Fear is often a buried emotion and totally subjective. John had not had a similar response. He had not remembered any situational details, only the fact that his baby was dead. Hence his response was of a more general anxiety yet not debilitating.

Inner feelings and outer expressions of emotions are linked and bodily signs of emotions often intensify emotional feelings. If an emotional facial expression promotes emotional experience, it follows that an inconsistent expression will reduce the intensity of the emotion.

So by appearing 'not bothered' this can diminish a feeling of being distressed. Some practitioners choose to cognitively deal with a stressor later when they are alone, especially if they are attempting to fulfil the requirements of their job. Some women are not prepared to show any signs of emotion and their response to receiving news may be very different to the midwife's expectations (based on her value system and clinical experience). The midwife may need to clarify that significant aspects of the news have been understood. The woman's micro expressions of real emotion often 'break through' her facial expressions and the midwife is likely to perceive her false smile, as exactly what it is. However if this is the woman's chosen way to cope with the situation, the midwife should respond with warmth and support, but cautious with touch (Pinel 2006).

Self-guides: the ideal self and the ought self

One of the most important aspects of self-regulation involves the way self-knowledge motivates behaviour towards important goals or standards and are referred to as self-guides, and are called the *ideal self* and the *ought self*. The ideal self is the person one would like to be. Self-discrepancies from the ideal self produce feelings of disappointment, sadness and dejection. The ought self is the person one considers one *should be* and this generally involves negative outcomes that people try to avoid and attempts to prevent failures lead to emotions of anger and agitation. Accomplishing 'ought goals' can produce feelings of relief and relaxation. See Case vignette 7.3

Case vignette 7.3

A natural birth was Heather's dream. For her it was part of being the mother she wanted to be and so it became part of her *ought self* and a '*should be*' outcome for her. She went on to have the birth she wanted and as a result felt a great sense of personal satisfaction and fulfilment.

Had the birth been different from that anticipated, Heather might have experienced a sense of loss and profound distress, which might have appeared to the midwife as totally disproportionate to the events that occurred because in accordance with the midwife's ought self, both mother and baby were alive and healthy. It is important for the midwife to understand what her *ought* agenda is and whether it is consistent with that of the woman's. In a hair salon, a good hairdresser finds out exactly what style the client wants and offers no hesitation in double-checking for meaning and understanding. A poor haircut will grow out in two weeks, but poor midwifery care can have long-term repercussions (Edworthy et al 2008, Leeds and Hargreaves 2008, White et al 2006). It takes a little bit more than a cursory glance at an extensive birth plan to know what this woman *really* wants. Such a response from the midwife communicates a certain type of arrogance that implies that she knows better.

Breastfeeding can be a challenging time for the self-concept because as a goal to be achieved, it may represent *an ideal* for one person and *an ought* for another. The 'ought' component may come from within or from an outside influence which may conflict with her own desires. In terms of the emotional impact of failing to attain the goal, what matters is the way each mother thinks about it. The midwife could ask 'is breastfeeding *a would like to achieve* or a *should achieve* event for you?' This type of question may only be asked if the woman is demonstrating some incongruence in her behaviour (see Chapter 5) and is often met with a need for more verbal explanation and exploration. The way questions are framed enables the woman to think about her situation and how she wants to proceed (Battersby 2009).

When applied to both women and midwives, negative effects of self-discrepancies can in extreme cases trigger emotions that lead to a cycle of sadness, anxiety, lowered self-esteem, even depression. Certain situations exaggerate awareness of discrepancies from self-guides and some people are highly aware of them. Self-fulfilling situations increase a person's self-awareness by directing attention to their inner standards and this heightens their awareness to whether they measure up to them. Some people are more focused than others on their internalised standards. Their increased awareness means that any negative self-related information leads to stronger feelings of distress and sadness (Deery 2009).

Self-presentations

Many people attempt to express their self-concept through their actions. Such self-expression confirms and reinforces the person's sense of self and also conveys it to other people. Their communication intention is to say, 'I am what I am'. By comparison, other people say, 'I am what you want me to be'. In the latter case, the person is creating a desirable impression; trying to shape the other person's impressions in order to gain power, influence or approval. Most people care about conveying a positive impression to others. Ingratiation (trying to convey the impression of being likeable) and self-promotion (trying to convey a message of competence) are the two most common goals of social interaction (Smith and Mackie 2007). Self-presentations are acting in a way that is consistent with the person's sense of the ideal. The self-presentation process has an effect on the private self and distinguishing the self-portrait from the self may become difficult as the person's performance becomes more polished and routine. What starts out as a mask, may eventually become the face (Simon and Trötschel 2008).

Defending the self from stresses and inconsistencies

The sense of self is a person's most valued possession and is treated that way. When events trigger the alarm system, there are either attempts to deal with what set off the alarm or efforts to change the way it makes the person feel. Lazarus (1991) sees stress as a transaction between a person and their environment. When faced with an event, the person will firstly appraise it as stressful or not and if so will further appraise it in terms of their personal resources (will I be able to cope?) which may include their social support networks and financial resources (see Chapter 8). A good person-environment fit results in the perception of little or low stress and a poor fit results in higher stress.

Types of stress

Eustress encompasses alertness, a creative tension that enables the person to function on a day-to-day basis and is seen as good stress because it comes from the word euphoria which means having a sense of wellbeing. Distress is seen as bad stress because it is derived from the Greek word *dys* which means bad. Life experiences tend to interact with each other and stressors can be short lived or long term.

What events are appraised as stressful?

According to Butler and Hope (2007) there are different types of stressful events and all are perceived differently but happen in the most important parts of one's life. An example may include:

- major changes like a pregnancy, marriage, separation, divorce, change of job
- loss of a friend or relative, giving up work to have children, losing one's job

- disruption to routine like having a new baby in the house, stopping smoking
- trouble and strife could represent arguments especially in a new relationship, relationship problems in general, financial difficulties, illness.

When events are ambiguous, a person may feel confused and do not know how to respond because they have difficulty in choosing a coping strategy. This can happen to a similar degree when events are uncontrollable. If a stressor can be predicted and controlled it is usually appraised as less stressful, for example public holidays like Christmas.

Many types of events create inconsistencies to the self-concept, for example an empty cot for a postnatal mother provides her with information that contradicts who and what she thought she would be. Events do not have to be negative to be inconsistent. Life changing events like marriage, or becoming a parent are joyous occasions in themselves but make for difficult changes in the self-concept. Ogden (2007) argues that early research studies on stress focused upon major life events, however later research has proposed that minor life events that arise from small but relentless frustrations and hassles of everyday life, the pressures of work, the boredom of routine, may together culminate in a negative way. All of these events call the sense of self into question. Smith and Mackie (2007) argue that threats to the self have effects beyond negative emotions and can adversely affect physical health. Positive emotions are strongly associated with better health. Coping strategies are undertaken to reduce negative consequences of self-threatening events.

The relationship between stress and coping

Carver (2007) asserts that coping with life stresses is part of normal existence, but asks what makes stressors particularly stressful? A single event may elevate, thrill and excite one person and be totally distressing to another. The event in itself does not change but totally depends upon the person's attitude or cognitive appraisal towards it and is defined as the *evaluative* process that determines *why* and *to what extent* a particular situation is perceived as stressful. First described by Lazarus and Folkman in 1984, they allied cognitive appraisal to coping and named three types of cognitive appraisal which is continuous and interdependent:

- primary appraisal distinguishes whether the threat is stressful or harmless
- secondary appraisal refers to the person's coping competencies at that time (consider 'it never rains but it pours')
- reappraisal refers to reassessment of the situation to ascertain whether the threatening situation has changed after the person's initial attempts to cope with it.

Coping is the use of cognitive and behavioural *strategies* that people use to manage both a stressful situation and the negative emotional reactions elicited by the event. In their model, Lazarus and Folkman (1984) distinguish two types of coping:

1. Problem or approach-focused coping strategies. Behaviour that directly deals with the stressor by acting to reduce or eliminate the risk of harmful consequences that might result from a stressful event. People attempt to reinterpret the event as non-threatening. They use:
   - *self-enhancing attributions* in which they take credit for their successes and attribute failure to external causes
   - *self-handicapping communications* prior to an anticipated event to enable the person to 'save face' should things not turn out as planned
   - *the seeking of support and information* to enable them to take control of their situation as blaming external causes only works momentarily

- *positive reappraisal tactics* to revisit the problem in order to reappraise it more favourably
- *logical analysis* of the problem through reflection
- *problem-solving actions* to think of the different ways to deal with the problem.

2. Emotion or avoidance-focused coping strategies. These do not focus on the stressful event itself, but on reducing the distressing emotional *reactions* to it. They are regarded as less effective ways of coping as they are more passive in style and as a consequence are more associated with mental health morbidity. People may use:

- *acceptance or resignation*. When events conspire to bring home failures and shortcomings, a common impulse is to flee rather than face the situation, so doing nothing is always an option.
- *the seeking of alternative rewards*. Escaping painful self-awareness through distraction may be as mundane as watching television. Alcohol consumption temporarily reduces self-awareness and 'drowning one's sorrows' may seem effective at the time in an attempt to temporarily blot out the uncomfortable consequences of self-discrepancy. Recreational drugs are used for the same reasons.
- *cognitive avoidance*. The use of selective inattention and forgetting is used to avoid the stressful information.
- *denial or repression of their true feelings*. This may be seen when there is incongruence between their physiological state and level of reported anxiety. When confronted with a stressor they say 'I'm fine' but their body is showing arousal. This suggests that although appraisal may be central to the stress response (Box 7.3) there may be some people in some situations that deny or repress their emotional response to a stressor.
- *re-affirmation* of the importance of other aspects of their life to off-set their sense of failure, uncertainty and stress in the area of concern.
- *self-expression* to work through the threat usually in the form of talking about their feelings which can help in making them feel more positive about themselves.
- *emotional discharge* which is 'taking it out on other people' when feeling angry or low in mood. Where professional power resides this could equate to bullying.
- *rumination* which is defined as unintentional preservative thoughts that occur in the absence of obvious external cues. An example is thinking about work out of hours when the midwife should be focused upon rest and leisure activities.

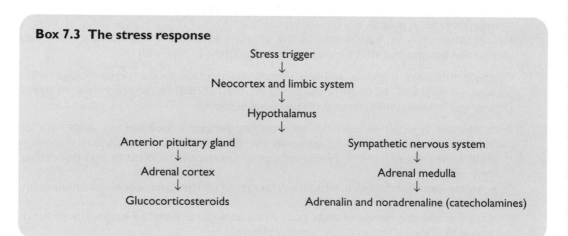

Box 7.3 The stress response

Stress trigger
↓
Neocortex and limbic system
↓
Hypothalamus
↓

Anterior pituitary gland   Sympathetic nervous system
↓   ↓
Adrenal cortex   Adrenal medulla
↓   ↓
Glucocorticosteroids   Adrenalin and noradrenaline (catecholamines)

Coping strategies and midwifery practice

Rumination: coping strategy or habit?

Butler and Hope (2007) believe that when people feel stressed, in a frenzy of anxious despair they constantly ruminate about all the things *they have to do* and all the things they *haven't yet done*. Living in the present moment enables the midwife to concentrate on what is happening at the present time, to do the task in hand effectively, then move on to the next one. A sense of achievement and satisfaction is thus created which replaces the temptation of starting too many tasks, but successfully completing little of quality and labelling oneself as being poorly organised or not coping. Rowe (2008) takes a feminist view and argues that when women denigrate themselves they feel anxious and guilty and a lot of time is taken up ruminating about themselves as not good enough or worrying about what other people think about them. She believes that they are trapped as prisoners in their own mind and as a process it becomes very wearing. They need to learn to get along with themselves, to relax and be comfortable in 'their own skin'.

Alfaraj et al (2009) report that this persistent recycling of negative thoughts can interfere with cognitive ability to problem-solve. Their research compared depressed and non-depressed pregnant women and found that the women who perceived rumination positively (thinking about my problems will help me feel better) and used it as a coping strategy, suffered a deterioration in their mental state. The researchers think this is an important finding, because by targeting women with positive beliefs about rumination, midwives may help them to develop more proactive coping strategies like talking about how they feel, instead of dwelling on the negative aspects of their life.

Cognitive avoidance and emotional discharge

In her study, Rodriguez (2009) found that in adult pregnant women, low pregnancy desire (an unplanned pregnancy) was significantly associated with the potential for physical child abuse. The women reported that they used avoidance-focused coping strategies, namely cognitive avoidance (I'm pregnant and I don't know what to do . . . and it is not going away) and emotional discharge (feelings of ambivalence to the unborn child because it (her baby) represents the source of her present problem). It is argued that pregnant women who express an ambivalent attitude towards their unborn baby may benefit from midwife support to discuss their feelings. This may help them to diminish their use of passive coping strategies in favour of more active approach-focused coping strategies. Such interventions would have the potential to facilitate and enhance mother–baby relationships (see Chapter 9).

Reflective activity

When you feel stressed, which coping strategies do you tend to rely upon more often? Think about a recent problem that has occupied your thoughts and reflect upon how you attempted to resolve it. To what extent did the strategies you employed, work for you?

Having knowledge of common coping strategies can help the midwife to understand how the people she cares for and works with, may use them to manage their stress. Reflection can help oneself to understand how different situations call for different approaches. Whether one considers the act of consuming large amounts of chocolate as a coping strategy is open to speculation, but does a certain degree of comfort eating represent a stressed society?

Multitasking has led to people having too much to do in each of the roles they play and has for some led to emotional exhaustion. On the other end of the stress continuum (see Fig. 7.2) there are people who have very little to do. Indeed some argue that not having a reason to get out of bed in the morning is more corrupting than having too much to do and is described as a totally demoralising state because the self-concept struggles with the reality of worthlessness (Marris 1991).

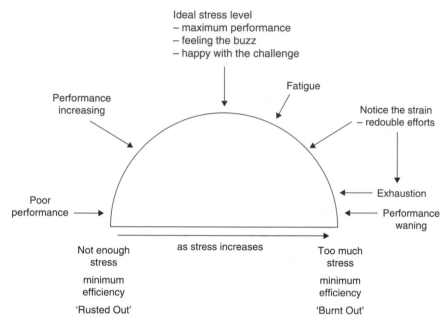

Figure 7.2 To illustrate the ideal stress level when performance is at its peak

The related states of fear, anxiety, stress and emotion

Fear: an emotional reaction to threat

According to Watt and Stuart (2008) fear is the emotional reaction to current threat. It is the motivating force for defensive behaviours, primarily to *protect* from harm. In contrast, aggressive behaviours have the primary function *to threaten and harm*. Most aggressive outbursts in people are over-reactions to real or perceived threat and they are appropriately viewed as defensive attack, not social aggression. When the body is exposed to threat the result is a cluster of physiological changes and according to Ogden (2007) fear can be long-lasting (chronic) psychological stress. Segerstrom and Miller (2004) in their meta-analysis of 300 studies found it was the kind of stress that was important. Acute (short-lived) stress can lead to improvements in immune function. By comparison, chronic stress such as caring for a handicapped child, experiencing different aspects of poverty, working long hours without adequate recuperation time, can adversely affect the more complex immune system processes. Stressed people often display changes in patterns of diet, exercise, sleep and drug use, all of which influence immune function (Pinel 2006).

Anxiety: preparing for threat

By comparison, anxiety tends to persist in the *absence* of any direct threat, but is the body's response to *perceived threat* that has not happened yet. It is a common physiologic correlate of stress and is adaptive as it motivates coping behaviours because it is telling the body to prepare. Anxiety has been traditionally seen as two common concepts. When it is a relatively permanent feature of a person's personality, it is considered a *trait*. When specific situations occur that create a transitory anxiety response, this is known as an *anxiety state*. Those people who have an existing anxiety trait may undergo further psychological distress during childbearing experiences and so have an increased anxiety state. Withdrawal may provoke a sense of feeling helpless when the person feels unable to gain any control over their situation because any actions they produce has little or no effect on the outcome. Watt and Stuart (2008) argue that for some people, the sensations of the physiological stress reactions such as tachycardia, sweating, nausea, dizziness and breathing difficulties, create anxiety in their own way. Such people have anxiety sensitivity and it's as if they 'turn up the volume' on these sensations. Less anxiety-sensitive people tend to reduce the volume, recognising these sensations to be normal, temporary and unpleasant, but otherwise harmless consequences of being in an anxiety state.

At what age can fear, stress and anxiety be experienced and learned?

A relatively new area of research suggests that fetal, neonatal and early life experiences of stress influence emerging emotional behaviour and associated cognitive problems (Glover and O'Connor 2006, Van den Berg et al 2005). The emphasis is on the development of the baby's brain, with implications for the amount of fetal stress/anxiety experienced in the uterus, the presence of any genetic vulnerabilities and when born, the degree of postnatal exposure to stressed parents. Glover and O'Connor (2006) argue that maternal symptoms of anxiety and depression are more common during pregnancy than in the postnatal period. Pregnancy is a period when relationships between parents may become strained and the incidence of domestic violence is known to be elevated. This research may have implications for the midwife, in providing a programme of anxiety reduction for the most anxious pregnant women, to safeguard the behaviour of their children.

Butler and Hope (2007) believe too that anxiety may be a learned behaviour related to the way the adult person attached to his or her parents in childhood. A person's model of self may range from little or no anxiety about rejection or abandonment to intense anxiety about rejection based on beliefs of personal unworthiness. A person's model of others could range from interpersonal trust to a mistrusting avoidance of others and discomfort with interpersonal closeness. Such behaviours need to be recognised as part of a person's learning history and not to be reinforced by careless attention to individual need (see Chapter 9 for a further discussion on attachment styles).

Anxiety and its effects on cognitive function

Cognition is about thinking, processing, problem solving and memory (see Chapter 1). Some of one's greatest fears are imagined more than realised. The thoughts people think and the kinds of things they say to themselves can either heighten or lessen their anxiety. Intrusive ruminations of previous experiences of anxiety include 'I'm a failure'; 'here we go again'; 'I can't do this'. Loss of concentration, feelings of panic and distress, even despair may be experienced. Consequently anxiety is a lonely place as no one else can really experience what the person is feeling and thinking. Lowering of self-esteem occurs when 'things keep going wrong' especially if associated with guilt or shame. The person may start to lose confidence in their ability to function in simple everyday events and as a result become indecisive and hypersensitive to criticism. Sometimes it is easier to avoid certain situations or people and much psychic energy can be utilised in devising excuses not to engage in interactions with others, thus their behaviour becomes disjointed. Emotional and cognitive fatigue may follow. Accident proneness is not uncommon as sleeping and eating patterns change. Interpersonal relationships may become strained. This correlates with decreased levels of effective communications and a poorer ability to problem-solve (Butler and Hope 2007). Anxiety may become so severe that it disrupts normal functioning and is then referred to as an anxiety disorder (see Chapter 4).

There are many examples in midwifery practice where the events are anxiety-provoking for all involved. Callam et al (1999) explore the extent to which mothers recall and understand information given to them at the time of preterm birth of a fragile baby requiring neonatal intensive care. They report that the shock of the event for many parents was so overwhelming it led to them using coping strategies in the form of denial and cognitive avoidance. It was reported that the midwife felt that she had given good information in a kind manner, while the mother recalled little of what was said and in some cases expressed anger about the professional involved. In the study, mothers reported that they were unable to understand information imparted to them because of its complexity and their capacity to listen was limited as they were more cognitively engaged in minimising the implications of what was being said to them. Midwives need to be sensitive to the coping strategies that each parent may be using and understand that as events unfold, they are likely to be distracted by profound nagging questions about whether their baby will live and if so, will he be brain damaged? They are continually engaged in a grieving process of adapting to new anxiety-provoking information and appreciation of what is said has to be set in this context. Stressing the importance of particular points, repetition of simple information, provision of a written summary may help, but the midwife must be prepared to answer the same question many times, knowing that her response is not being fully attended to and on many occasions there are no definitive answers to highly significant yet unrelenting questions (see Box 7.1).

Self-efficacy and coping

Bandura (1977) argues that self-efficacy is the extent to which people engage in self-regulation and thus emerge as influential social agents and this notion is highly related to their beliefs or expectations about their ability to control their environment and achieve important goals. The higher perceived is self-efficacy, the stronger one's effort to attain a desired goal, even in the face of obstacles or failure. It is also important to note that self-efficacy expectations are not general beliefs about control. Rather, they are domain-specific perceptions of one's own ability to perform behaviours that lead to the attainment of a desired end-state.

According to Bandura (1997) there are four main sources of self-efficacy:

1. Personal experience of success or mastery
2. Observing effects produced by the actions of others such as parents, peers, teachers. Surrounding oneself with competent social models transmits knowledge for skill and strategy development
3. Social persuasion and encouragement from respected others
4. Modifying one's stress response. Anxiety, stress, fear and fatigue all deleteriously impact on self-efficacy. A positive mood enhances perceived self-efficacy whereas a negative mood diminishes it. By interpreting one's physical arousal as something positive, one can enhance mood and feel energised. However, such self-regulation processes call for a high degree of consistency and commitment and may become depleted with over-use. The person can become cognitively exhausted and will need to rest and recuperate (Simon and Trötschel 2008).

A person's degree of hardiness influences their appraisal of potential stressors and the resulting stress response. It involves a personal feeling of control, a desire to accept challenges and commitment, to see things through. Accordingly a feeling of being in control may contribute to the process of primary appraisal. Their feelings of mastery may reflect their sense of control over their stress response. Being successful is a strong motivator for further challenge. However, Williams et al (2008) argue that self-efficacy theory may not necessarily be a useful predictor in certain situations and in their study they questioned whether women who were attending antenatal education classes, with a perceived heightened sense of self-efficacy, were able to make choices about analgesia in labour. Given the uncertainty of the hospital environment and the unique nature of labour, even the most motivated mother may opt for epidural. Williams et al (2008) take issue with antenatal education and claim that it is based upon non-specific generalisations and perceived social expectations and does not provide enough clearly expressed contemporary, accurate information. They argue that targeting women's beliefs about different medications will impact upon their plans for analgesia to facilitate their decision-making processes. They further emphasise the need to include people close to them in their discussions. Attempting to make such important choices in active labour is not appropriate and renders the woman more susceptible to persuasive communications (see Chapter 5) and disappointment with herself if she succumbs to what she may perceive as the easy option. How easy is it to think the body into a course of action when birth is for many, couched in such a negative mindset?

In confident coping, Chambers (2009) believes that each person needs to ask how they view their stress situation. Does their emotional response to an event need to change so that it no longer creates distress and anxiety? By changing the attitude to the object or event, the picture changes; it is perceived in a different way. In order to change attitude, one needs to also ask *where* one's attitudes come from? Are they derived from past events that have little bearing on coping with life in the present? Defence mechanisms, barriers and labels (which people apply to themselves), may be remnants of previous coping, but can act as prisms that colour perception and predispose the person to react in a particular way; but is that way still relevant? Confident coping also calls for asking for help from others. People often think that a sign of not coping is to ask others for help and support. Above all, confident coping is about accepting one's own humanity. People are not programmed for perfection so learning to forgive oneself is vital and is influential in learning to forgive others. People who are judgemental and hard on themselves are often the same with others (Schafer 2000).

The psychology of giving and receiving help

According to Bierhoff (2008) receiving and being seen to receive help is not always a positive experience. Receiving help may burden the person with negative implications of weakness, even inferiority, and it can make them indebted to the helper. It can be particularly irritating to the recipient if they do not need the help on offer. The help, whether welcomed or not, establishes a debt to the helper and the recipient's freedom of choice is restricted and this may arouse a need for the recipient to restore it. The helper benefits from the notion that giving help is regarded as a desirable and fair thing to do and makes one feel good. It is acknowledged that helping as part of professional obligation is distinguished from more general altruism which is motivated by compassion, but people are more likely to show a helping attitude if they are in a positive mood, respond empathically and have an internal locus of control for that situation. It is therefore important that midwives give help sensitively when it is needed and are careful not to threaten the woman's self-esteem. It is difficult to support another's sense of empowerment if there is a reminder of the midwife's superiority.

Control and coping

Feelings of helplessness and/or powerlessness often equate to a person's sense of control (Dryden 2009). It is argued that if a person feels in control they will be less anxious. Rotter (1966) asked the question 'what controls events in people's everyday lives?' To answer this, he produced a self-administered questionnaire comprising 23 pairs of opposed statements and then devised a bipolar continuum of locus of control made up of internal and external extremes. The word locus means where the person's perception of control resides. A person with a perceived internal locus of control believes that what happens to them is as a consequence of their own doing. They believe that people's misfortunes result from the mistakes they make. A person with a perceived external locus of control believes that luck, fate, chance or other people and events, control most of the aspects of their life. Rotter (1966) believes that most people orientate around the middle of the continuum and offers the view that people with an internal locus of control are more likely to cope effectively with their anxiety. Indeed the perception or mere possibility of personal control is thought to produce an internally oriented state which may lead to a sense of decreased powerlessness.

Hospitalisation can be seen as an externalising event because when a person enters into a role-set like mother and midwife, the woman hopes that her named midwife will offer appropriate information, support and acceptance, a principle which also apples to student midwives and their mentors (Pryjmachuk and Richards 2008). Midwives are power people and can turn a confident woman into an anxious 'child'. Women do not know the hospital systems, often have to ask for things and therefore feel dependent. They may be distressed, frightened or in pain and may not understand all that is said to them. These factors can be modified by emphasising client self-reliance and informed choice and consent, but it is largely dependent upon how these concepts are communicated to them. To empower the mother to make informed choices means that the midwife must render some of her own power. This usually takes the form of midwifery/medical information, sharing the way systems work, keeping the client informed of progress and asking permission to give care (Nursing and Midwifery Council 2008). Sometimes it is difficult for midwives to see themselves as powerful in situations where they feel anxious and uncertain about their own professional role and there is a tendency for them not to relinquish any of their professional power but use it to reinforce their own perception of control in themselves. In this situation, the woman with an internal locus of control (my world is predictable and controllable by my own actions) may struggle to perceive personal control and may not be able to negotiate the conditions that enable her to cope effectively. The woman who perceives an external locus of control (health and illness are the responsibility of powerful others like doctors and midwives) may be quite satisfied with the midwife who makes decisions for her. Even when the woman is given the opportunity to make a choice, some will choose not to do so. Some cannot choose what they desire. The way women express themselves may give the midwife some indication of where their locus of control may reside *at that time*. Therefore the perception of control is highly subjective and can change over situations and time and coupled with the person's sense of self-efficacy, some situations can be extremely anxiety-provoking and may also be affected by the midwife's own self-efficacy in being able to offer psychological support, encouragement and empowerment.

Fear, anxiety and birthing, not a winning combination

According to Raphael-Leff (2005) a woman in labour has a heightened awareness of non-verbal cues; the tone rather than the words, sensing brusque roughness of touch or a disparaging glance, picking up vibrations of anxiety, sensing acceptance or disapproval. Such emotions may tune into her unresolved conflicts at a time when she is feeling particularly vulnerable and extra sensitive. Concurrent emotions such as anxiety, panic, uncertainty and fatigue may affect the way she perceives discomfort and pain, influenced strongly by cultural norms and her expectations. Some women have few experiences of feeling safe or soothed and are not able to do this for themselves. They have made anxiety and self-blaming into an art form and need others to show them how.

How pain is perceived depends on how the person has structured meaning for that experience. Many women can feel isolated, even if accompanied by their choice of companion. The contractions are so unfamiliar they can engender a sense of bewilderment and given their uniqueness can create psychological isolation as no other person, including the woman will experience what she is facing at this point in time. Hodnett et al (2008) argues that an anxious tense, 'out of control' woman thrashing about and crying with pain during early labour can be one of the greatest challenges to the intrapartum midwife. There is a temptation to think that 'her pain is not as bad as she thinks' which reflects the midwife's failure to appreciate the subjectivity of pain. The woman's pain is as bad as *she* thinks because her pain is exactly as she perceives it. The midwife may instead ask 'how can I make a difference in the pain experience of this woman? The reception a woman receives when arriving on the labour ward may affect the course of her labour. See Case vignette 7.4.

Case vignette 7.4

Elsa thought she was in labour and had telephoned the hospital to be told that she should stay at home and occupy herself with simple tasks. On the third day of being in this state, when her discomfort became, in her own words, 'too much' she came to the hospital. The midwife's haughtiness about her pre-labour (sometimes known as false labour) and the timing of when she had come to hospital shocked her. She felt foolish and now fears returning to hospital as she may meet the same midwife or others like her.

The humiliation of being spoken to in such an uncaring way and then being sent home like a naughty child, is damaging to the woman's self-esteem. It is argued by Hodnett et al (2008) that when labour does eventually occur, women like Elsa are more likely to experience more difficult labours caused by stress and fatigue, which often lead to instrumental or operative delivery.

When a woman is in early labour, it is so important to get her off to a good start. How she starts labour often dictates how she continues it. If she is not in active labour she needs distraction, support and reassurance rather than care per se. The midwife can assess the woman through observation of her muscle tension (wincing or relaxing during contractions), her breathing pattern (smooth or strained), her facial expression (calm or anxious) and her vocalisations (quiet sighs or grunting cries). Her attitude of acceptance to the contractions (it's here that's great) is a positive coping-related response compared to dread (it's coming to get me) which is a distress-related response (negative cognitive appraisal). The midwife can teach the mother to use positive coping strategies or reinforce her already established positive attitude.

When a woman starts to feel anxious, fearful, self-conscious or threatened, the amygdala (see Fig. 7.1), which is designed for survival, responds by preventing the birth. It rapidly triggers the release of catecholamines and cortisol (see Fig. 7.2) which alert her body to run, fight, freeze or submit. Blood is sent to her brain and skeletal muscles and is redirected away from the uterus, thus there is less blood flow to the placental site and the fetal tissues may become poorly oxygenated (hypoxia) and start to accumulate carbon dioxide (herpercapnia). Catecholamines are incompatible with oxytocin, therefore uterine contractions reduce in number and duration.

Hence the birth has been successfully slowed so that birth does not take place only when the threatening situation no longer exists.

In the care setting, this physiological response is usually referred to as failure to progress and brings with it its own threats (see Chapter 8). So fear, muscle tension and pain are the components of a labour that has been disrupted. The midwife's task is to reduce threat as much as possible to allow labour to continue (Dick-Read 2004). What constitutes threat will vary for each woman. Anger, fear, panic, anxiety, disgust are emotions that can be triggered by the fear of, or experience of pain, bad or mixed memories of a previous birth (Kitzinger 2009), her baby in distress, memories of sexual abuse. These are cognitive representations that will affect her ability to relax.

Buunk and Dijkstra (2008) assert that women who want to be cared for, innately cue midwives by their own facial expressions, tone of voice and touch, that they are willing to respond. In a reciprocal way women in labour will seek out attachment figures because of their kind face, the warmth and tone of their voice and gentle touch to soothe and dampen their threat system. However, many women are not in a position to choose their midwife and she may have to endure her labour with a midwife who appears unsympathetic to her needs. Women who have attended Hypnobirthing classes or are intending to use aromatherapy or waterbirth in their labour, need to be cared for by appropriately trained midwives who can support them in a confident reassuring manner (DH 2008).

Use of silence and being quiet is an important aspect of care in labour (see Chapter 6). Stimulating the woman's neocortex by drawing her into discussions that expect her to make decisions is undesirable. It is often argued that because she has an effective epidural block she will be able to cognitively engage. Informed consent is an important part of care but is counterproductive in active labour. If she is able to totally concentrate on her self she will be able to block out the environment (and the people in it). The midwife needs to be able to facilitate this philosophy and actively inhibit any distractions that are interfering with the woman's primitive instincts of needing to be left alone (Odent 1986). This approach has implications for fathers that their presence may inhibit the labour if they are not fully educated in what their role entails. Johnson (2002) believes there can be serious repercussions for fathers as high stress levels are often reflected in their negative feelings about being pressured to be present at the birth, coupled with unfulfilled role expectations. It is regrettable that post-traumatic stress disorder has been an unfortunate consequence of being present in the labour room, for a small but significant number of fathers (see Chapter 3).

Work stress and anxiety

Case vignette 7.4 appears to be critical of the midwife, but she may be caring for too many women, and the addition of yet another one needing her time and emotional energy creates a real sense of fear and panic in her. Unfortunately her manner sets the tone for Elsa's experience. Dykes (2009) reports that midwives feel that the volume of work they are expected to do is a strong contributor of stress and crucially involves the conditions that affect personal performance. Some lack job autonomy which involves control over the speed or nature of decisions made within the role. Poor relationships in the workplace and role ambiguity create tensions and directly affect social support systems. Emotional support involves trust between colleagues and social cohesion. Instrumental support involves the provision of extra resources and assistance. Job satisfaction may be affected as productivity falls and accident rates increase. Contact with anxious women and their partners can be stressful and the more contact time they have with them, the more anxious and emotionally exhausted the midwife may become.

Coping strategies in the workplace may include:

- psychological detachment-only engaging in a task-orientated or physical way with little use of empathy
- physical distancing – avoiding the woman's room or care area
- social intellectualisation – the inappropriate use of jargon that is used to suppress discussion or any form of verbal interaction.

Short- or long-term absenteeism may be a coping strategy as the midwife feels she cannot continue to function in her current state.

Marris (1991) argues that the qualities of good social relationships and positive experiences of attachment are essentially the same because they involve the features of predictability, responsiveness, intelligibility, supportiveness and reciprocity of commitment. With stress (and sometimes failure) come widespread insecurity and the more powerful members of the work team may seek to control the uncertainty in the behaviour of others without diminishing their own freedom. This leads to an enhanced tendency to subordinate and marginalise others in the interest of one's own greater security. Thus in a group where one dominant person is stressed everyone experiences the fallout. This inequality of control tends to displace the burden of uncertainty onto the weakest and profoundly influences the circumstances of attachment, leaving the most vulnerable at most risk of lowered mood, helplessness and grief.

In governing their relationships with others, people need to adopt the first principle of reciprocity of commitment, predictability and respect in order to protect the unique structures of meaning and attachment, which makes life worthwhile for everyone. Personal relationships are one's deepest need, so creating a world in which people dare attach, is vital for healthy survival (Marris 1991). Leaders of work teams need to emphasise the importance of the emotional dimensions of people's need and direct their skills to cherish and nurture the midwives in their care so that they, the midwives, can be free of the ravaging and debilitating effects of fear, anxiety and stress, to feel confident to offer emotional support to the women and families in their care.

Conclusion

Clearly a number of factors influence stress, fear and anxiety that arise from within the person and within their environment. In the midwifery setting, women, their partners and families are continually being challenged by different stressors and how they respond will vary based upon their life experiences, cultural background, gender and many other salient issues pertinent to them at the time. The way they have constructed their self-concept, how they perceive their ideal self, sense of self-efficacy and self-esteem, will impact upon the type and degree of physiological stress response they will experience, mediated through their cognitive appraisal of impending or actual threat. Add to this mix the midwife and the multi-agency team. They bring the same conceptual frameworks of self, but with different notions and constructions of threat.

The psychology of providing high quality woman-centred care from the base of a team is demanding because the midwife has to satisfy the demands of her own self–schema, protect her self-esteem, support the mother's self-esteem, render some of her control to the mother in order to empower her and work cohesively with the team. The stressed and anxious midwife in attempting to be congruent and empathic may struggle with the inconsistency. Her cognitive function may be affected and is often first noticed at the communication level. Her tone of voice may be more shrill; her facial expression less relaxed and more allied to one of anguish. Thus the 'amygdala sensitive' mother will be cued by the midwife and then she in turn, may start to feel uneasy.

Midwives need to know and understand what triggers a stress response in them. They need to consider their constructed self-guides and ask what they consider is their 'ought' and 'should' agendas. They need to question whether their coping strategies are approach-focused or avoidance-focused (Lazarus and Folkman 1984) and whether they are and remain effective. Coping is an important element in maintaining wellbeing and regular reappraisal of one's approach may bring about important insights into managing fear, anxiety and stress in the workplace.

Summary of key points

- The self-concept is each person's most valued possession and when it is threatened through the process of cognitive appraisal, the use of coping strategies are used to preserve its consistency.

- The limbic system is linked to primitive functions of survival and negative cognitive appraisals will stimulate the amygdala to trigger a fear response. Facial expressions and tone of voice are particularly registered, alongside memories of past experiences.

- Women in labour are 'amygdala sensitive' and the cycle of fear, muscle tension and pain can be easily triggered by a brusque tone and/or sour face. By using soothing behaviours, the midwife can dampen the woman's threat system.

- The aura of tension that surrounds a stressed and anxious person is easily transferred to another person. A stressed midwife can stop a labour. An anxious woman may threaten a midwife's dwindling emotional resources to cope.

- The receiving of significant news is an example of how the woman's unique threat system can be stimulated. Within seconds, the combined effects of the limbic and autonomic nervous system may render her unable to coherently respond. News is neutral and in any situation of giving news, the woman's physiological response is always an unknown.

- Pregnancy stress is associated with fetal stress, which is thought to adversely affect neurological and behavioural development in the baby.

- The perception of self-efficacy is diminished by stress, anxiety and fear.

- Where work stress is a dominant cultural feature, the more powerful can marginalise, divide and disempower the less assertive members of the team. As coping strategies become exhausted, absenteeism may, for some people, be the only option left available.

References

Alfaraj, A.M.A., Spada, M.M., Nikcevic, A.V., Puffett, A. and Meer, S. (2009) Positive beliefs about rumination in depressed and non-depressed pregnant women: a preliminary investigation. *Journal of Reproductive and Infant Psychology*, 27(1): 54–60.

Bandura, A. (1997) *Self-efficacy: the exercise of control*. New York: Freeman.

Bandura, A. (1977) Self-efficacy: toward a unifying theory of behavioural change, *Psychological Review*, 84(2): 191–215.

Battersby, S. (2009) Midwives, infant feeding and emotional turmoil. In: B. Hunter, R. Deery (eds) *Emotions in Midwifery and Reproduction*. London: Palgrave Macmillan.

Bem, D.J. (1967) Self perception: An alternative interpretation of cognitive dissonance phenomena. *Psychological Review*, 74: 183–200.

Bierhoff, H.W. (2008) Pro-social behaviour. In: M. Hewstone, W. Stroebe and K. Jonas (eds) *Introduction to Social Psychology. A European perspective*. Oxford: Blackwell.

British Association for Counselling and Psychotherapy (2009) What is counselling? www.bacp.co.uk, accessed 12 June 09.

Butler, G. and Hope, T. (2007) *Manage your Mind. The mental fitness guide*. Oxford: Oxford University Press.

Buunk, A.P. and Dijkstra, P. (2008) Affiliation, attraction and close relationships. In: M. Hewstone, W. Stroebe and K. Jonas (eds) *Introduction to Social Psychology. A European perspective*, 4th edn. Oxford: Blackwell.

Callam, R.M., Lambrenos, K., Cox, A.D. and Weindling, A.M. (1999) Maternal appraisal of information given around the time of preterm delivery. *Journal of Reproductive and Infant Psychology*, 17(3): 267–80.

Carver, C.S. (2007) Stress, coping, and health. In: H.S. Friedman, R.C. Silver (eds) *Health Psychology*. Oxford: Oxford University Press.

Chambers, M. (2009) Anxiety. In: A. Gasper, G. McEwing, J. Richardson (eds) *Foundation Skills for Caring*. London: Palgrave Macmillan.

Deery, R. (2009) Community midwifery 'performances' and the presentation of self. In: B. Hunter, R. Deery (eds) *Emotions in Midwifery and Reproduction*. London: Palgrave Macmillan.

Department of Health (2008) *High Quality Care For All: NHS next stage review final report* (Darzi Review). www.dh.gov.uk, accessed 26 June 09.

Dick-Read, G. (2004) *Childbirth without Fear: the principles and practice of natural childbirth*. London: Pinter and Martin Books.

Dryden, W. (2009) *Understanding Emotional Problems*. London: Routledge.

Dykes, F. (2009) 'No time to care': midwifery work on postnatal wards in England. In: B. Hunter and R. Deery (eds) *Emotions in Midwifery and Reproduction*. New York: Palgrave Macmillan.

Edworthy, Z., Chasey, R. and Williams, H. (2008) The role of schema and appraisals in the development of post-traumatic stress symptoms following birth. *Journal of Reproductive and Infant Psychology*, 26(2): 123–38.

Glover, V. and O'Connor, T. (2006) Maternal anxiety: its effect on the fetus and the child. *British Journal of Midwifery*, 14(11): 663–7.

Goffman, E. (1990) *The Presentation of Self in Everyday Life*. Harmondsworth: Penguin.

Hodnett, E.D., Stremler, R., Willan, A.R. et al and the SELAN trial group (2008) Effect on birth outcomes of a formalised approach to care in hospital labour assessment units: international, randomized controlled trial. www.bmj.com/cgi/content/full/337:a1021, accessed 07 June 09.

Johnson, M.P. (2002) The implications of unfulfilled expectations and perceived pressure to attend the birth on men's stress levels following birth attendance: a longitudinal study. *Journal of Psychosomatic Obstetrics and Gynaecology*, 23: 173–82.

Kitzinger, S. (2009) *Birth Crisis*, 2nd edn. London: Routledge.

Lazarus, R.S. (1991) *Emotion and Adaptation*. New York: Oxford University Press.

Lazarus, R.S. and Folkman, S. (1984) *Stress, Appraisal and Coping*. New York: Springer-Verlag.

Leeds, L. and Hargreaves, I. (2008) The psychological consequences of childbirth. *Journal of Reproductive and Infant Psychology*, 26(2): 108–22.

Marris, P. (1991) The social construction of uncertainty. In: C.M. Parkes, J. Stevenson-Hinde, P. Marris (eds) *Attachment across the Life Cycle*. London: Routledge.

Nursing and Midwifery Council (2008) *The Code*. London: NMC.

Odent, M. (1986) *Primal Health*. London: Hutchinson Press.

Ogden, J. (2007) *Health Psychology*, 4th edn. Maidenhead: McGraw-Hill.

Pinel, J.P.J. (2006) *Biopsychology*, 6th edn. London: Pearson.

Pryjmachuk, S. and Richards, D.A. (2008) Predicting stress in pre-registration midwifery students attending a university in Northern England. *Midwifery*, 24: 108–22.

Raphael-Leff, J. (2005) *Psychological Processes of Childbearing*, 4th edn. Kings Lynn: The Anna Freud Centre.

Rodriguez, C.M. (2009) Coping style as a mediator between pregnancy desire and child abuse potential: a brief report. *Journal of Reproductive and Infant Psychology*, 27(1): 61–9.

Rotter, J.B. (1966) Generalized expectancies of internal versus external control of reinforcement. *Psychological Monographs*, 30(1): 1–26.

Rowe, D. (2008) *What Should I Believe?* London: Routledge.

Segerstrom, S.C. and Miller, G.E. (2004) Psychological stress and the human immune system: A meta-analytic study of 30 years of inquiry. *Psychological Bulletin*, 130: 601–30.

Schafer, W. (2000) *Stress Management for Wellness*. London: Thomson Wadsworth.

Simon, B. and Trötschel, R. (2008) Self and social identity. In: M. Hewstone, W. Stroebe, K. Jonas (eds) *Introduction to Social Psychology. A European perspective*, 4th edn. Oxford: Blackwell.

Smith, E.R. and Mackie, D.M. (2007) *Social Psychology*, 3rd edn. Hove: Psychological Press.

Smith, J.A. (1999) Identity development during the transition to motherhood: an interpretive phenomenological analysis. *Journal of Reproductive and Infant Psychology*, 17(3): 281–99.

Van den Berg, B.R., Mulder, E.J., Mennes, M. and Glover, V. (2005) Antenatal maternal anxiety and stress and the neurobehavioural development of the fetus and child: links and possible mechanisms. A review. *Neuroscience Biobehavioural Review*, 29(2): 237–58.

Watt, M.C. and Stuart, S.H. (2008) *Overcoming the Fear of Fear. How to reduce anxiety sensitivity*. Oakland, Canada: New Harbinger Publications.

White, T., Matthey, S., Boyd, K. and Barnett, B. (2006) Postnatal depression and post-traumatic stress after childbirth: prevalence, course and co-occurrence. *Journal of Reproductive and Infant Psychology*, 24(2): 107–20.

Williams, C.E., Povey, R.C. and White, D.G. (2008) Predicting women's intentions to use pain relief medication during childbirth using the theory of planned behaviour and self efficacy theory. *Journal of Reproductive and Infant Psychology*, 26(3): 168–79.

Woolsey, T.A., Hanaway, J. and Gado, M.H. (2008) *The Brain Atlas*. New Jersey: Wiley.

Annotated further reading

Pardey, D. (2007) *Superseries. Managing Stress in the Workplace*. London: Pergamon Flexible Learning.

A useful workbook that is person friendly with activities to complete.

Pargman, D. (2006) *Managing Performance Stress*. London: Routledge.

A detailed text about focuses on cognitive processing and reframing the stressor.

Website

www.easierbirth.co.uk

8 | Psychosocial support

Chapter contents

Introduction

Chapter aims

What is psychosocial support?

Dimensions of support

What does the evidence say?

Continuity of carer: is it important to women?

Type of care giver – who should support
   women during labour?

Models of good practice

Role of the midwife

Conclusion

Summary of key points

References

Annotated further reading

Useful websites

Introduction

For centuries women have given birth supported by others, usually wise women with prior experience of pregnancy and childbirth. However, in Western cultures, the shift from home to hospital as the ubiquitous place of birth has signalled a 21st-century phenomenon: the demise of such cultural practices and traditions that ensured women during pregnancy and childbirth received continuous support from their female relatives. The nature of impersonal hospital settings means that the quality of support women receive in contemporary midwifery practice is quite variable. This is also compounded by the structure, culture and organisation of maternity care in the NHS within the UK as well as the national shortage of midwives. Yet, longitudinal studies of support during pregnancy, coupled with research focusing on the evaluation of one-to-one care in labour, have highlighted the good outcomes and benefits of this intervention for mothers and babies (Hodnett et al 2007, Wiggins et al 2004, Sandall et al 2001, Murray et al 2000, Oakley et al 1996). Furthermore, in the context of normality, the World Health Organization (1999) specifically states that the midwife is the health professional best placed to support women as well as provide the most appropriate and cost effective care. Murray et al (2000: 254) stress that every effort should be made to enable midwives to prioritise care to give continuous support to women. This is particularly crucial during labour when midwives can find themselves juggling care for women alongside performing non-essential or 'less ineffective activities'. The goal of this chapter is to take a critical look at the concept of support and how it may benefit women and their families emotionally, psychologically and socially.

Chapter aims

- To provide an operational definition for the term psychosocial support

- To identify the evidence base in order to discuss the different dimensions of support provided by the midwife, the doula or the partner

- To discuss psychosocial support as a major determinant of health and wellbeing for women during the childbearing continuum

- To highlight the skills needed by midwives to provide effective support for women and families

- To identify models of good practice

What is psychosocial support?

Finding a standard definition is not an easy feat, but it is important in practice to have an operational definition of the term **support** if the concept is to be fully understood. Student midwives as well as midwives will be familiar with its use by simply reflecting on how support is employed in aspects of their day-to-day lives. Support means different things to different people. To clarify meaning and understanding, the reader is invited to work through the activity outlined in Box 8.1.

Box 8.1 Reflective activity to explore the meaning of support

Examine the following statements and provide a simple definition of your understanding of the concept **support** and in doing so consider why the concept is important to emotional health/wellbeing.

1. She has plenty of social support.
2. She is receiving financial support from her parents
3. Her partner provides no child support
4. She is on life support
5. IT support is needed to update the computer program
6. His story supports his claim
7. The evidence supports current practice
8. She had the courage to challenge the organisation and support her colleague.
9. The essay is well supported by the literature
10. The support group was invaluable to her establishing and maintaining breastfeeding
11. She was supported in labour by leaning against the bath
12. The mechanism of midwifery supervision is a legal framework that provides support for practising midwives
13. She was supported by her manager to attend the workshop.

It is recognised that optimal outcomes for mothers and babies are achieved when women are provided with quality care from skilled and knowledgeable midwives who can communicate, collaborate and engage the help and support of other members of the multiprofessional team when there is a clear indication to do so (Homer et al 2001, Sandall et al 2001). Ideally this should be through schemes that ensure continuity of care with carer and supports a model of care provided by a midwife that the woman knows and trusts (Page 2003, Sandall et al 2001). Support is synonymous with a number of words as depicted in Box 8.2. The list is not exhaustive and the reader is encouraged to add to the list.

Box 8.2 Some alternative words to the term support

bolster; maintain; help; encourage; aid; backup; advocate; champion; sustain; corroborate; substantiate; defend; reassuring; vouch for; strengthen

---

As can be seen from completing the activity in Box 8.1 and reflecting on the words synonymous with the notion of support in Box 8.2, it is a complex and subjective concept to define. For the purpose of this chapter psychosocial support is defined as the social interaction between a woman and significant other – partner, relative, friend, doula or healthcare professional such as the midwife – that has a buffering effect, so that the help provided is instrumental in promoting self-determination and assisting the woman to cope in a positive manner. The relationship should be one based on mutual respect and trust in order that the woman feels safe and protected. Supporting women should nurture, sustain, provide empathetic understanding in the form of praise, reciprocity, encouragement and be genuine. Finally it should fulfil the woman's informational, physical and emotional needs.

Dimensions of support

Hodnett et al (2007) identify four dimensions to support during labour: emotional support, informational support, physical support and advocacy as illustrated in Figure 8.1.

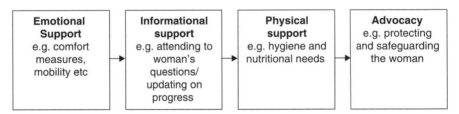

Figure 8.1 Dimensions of support. Adapted from Hodnett et al (2007)

What does the evidence say?

Psychological and emotional wellbeing are regarded as prerequisites that enable parents and their children to evolve into socially and emotionally well-adjusted and caring citizens, culminating in a healthier nation (Department of Health [DH] 2004). A healthy and positive approach to mental health is a fundamental start any parent can provide for their child. This investment, Vimpani (2000) states, requires sound social support network structures or what he refers to as 'social capital'. From the evidence base, both nationally and internationally, there is firm acknowledgement of the significant public health contribution midwives make in providing support for women throughout pregnancy, labour and postpartum (DH 2004, 2007,

2008, Lewis 2007, WHO 1999). This extends not only to meeting the physical needs of women but also to fulfilling their psychosocial and emotional needs. The general care of women, provision of health education/promotion, informational support for them and their families during the course of pregnancy, labour and the puerperium are important. Table 8.1 highlights some of the pivotal work undertaken to build a critical mass of evidence around support in pregnancy and childbirth.

Support also extends to the recognition of deviations from normality and making appropriate referrals to other members of the multiprofessional team on a needs basis. These fundamental elements of the midwife's role are clearly spelt out by the Nursing and Midwifery Council (NMC 2004) and International Confederation of Midwives (ICM 2005). Hunter and Deery's (2009) central critique on 'emotion work' (see Chapter 6) challenges the way in which

Table 8.1 Psychosocial support: useful evidence

Evidence	Type of study	Practice implications
Oakley et al (1996) social support in pregnancy **Strength of the evidence: level 2**	Longitudinal study randomised and non-blinded (N=509 women)	Additional support and continuity of care benefit disadvantage groups by improving birth weight and bringing about behavioural change.
Hodnett et al (2007) Continuous support in labour **Strength of the evidence: level 1**	Cochrane database of systematic review of 6 randomised controlled trials (RCTs) (N=13,391 women)	Highlights importance of continuous support of birth companion of woman's choice during labour, especially from doula in achieving normality and reducing intervention. Other areas addressed • Type of care giver support • Timing of continuous support • Interventions e.g. use of EFM and pain relief
Wiggins et al (2004) postpartum social support **Strength of the evidence: level 2**	Longitudinal RCT (N=731 women)	Postpartum social support in the form of 'listening visits' by health visitors may improve some aspects of emotional well-being.
Sandall et al (2001) Evaluation of the Albany midwifery practice **Strength of the evidence: level 2**	Data collection methods included: focus groups, questionnaires, interviews, analysis of routine audit data and document analysis 447 women selected at random (N=231 responded to the survey)	Higher rates of: • homebirths • vaginal births • breastfeeding Lower rates of interventions e.g.: • LSCS • Pharmacological methods of pain relief • episiotomies • inductions
McCourt et al (1998) One-to-one care in labour **Strength of the evidence: level 2**	Prospective comparative longitudinal cohort study using both quantitative and qualitative methodology: self completion questionnaires, interviews and focus groups (728 women in study group & 675 women in control group)	Women demonstrated a preference for continuity of care with known carer and seem to make a more positive adaptation to the mothering role. This and the penultimate study proves that RCTs are not always the most appropriate methodology for women and midwives.

student midwives are socialised and educated as they journey through their pre-registration programme in the UK, pointing out that students are driven to fulfil a competency framework, a requirement of the NMC, but at the expense of time being spent developing a sound comprehension of the emotional task involved in supporting women and helping to meet their psychological needs.

Continuity of carer: is it important to women?

The benefits of continuous support during labour is well documented (Hodnett et al 2007, Martis 2007, McCourt et al 1998) and includes a strong likelihood of women realising a spontaneous vaginal birth with a shorter labour and reduced need for medical intervention including pharmacological means of analgesia. What is less transparent in the literature is whether all dimensions of continuity of carer matters to women. Green et al's (2000) literature review reveals the different interpretations and limited definitions of continuity of carer, making it a challenging concept. They conclude that there is no evidence to support the claim that women were more satisfied with their care when cared for in labour by a midwife they had already met compared to those women who had no prior contact with their midwife. The researchers state that what matters most to women is kind, reliable or consistent care from skilled and trusted midwives that make women feel safe. Nonetheless, the evidence is clear, women who perceive psychosocial support during pregnancy and childbirth as a positive intervention are more likely to be satisfied with their birth experience, which is important as they embrace their responsibilities of early motherhood, as illustrated in Verity's story (Chapter 6).

Challenges

Page (2003) identifies some of the challenges of providing continuity of care with carer for midwives. These include 24 hour on call, 7 days per week (excluding holidays), a pattern that can prove tiring and stressful even for the most keen and committed midwife. Despite these challenges, Page (2003) points out that continuity of care means that the midwife is truly with woman, working 'with the woman' rather than 'doing to or for the woman'.

Type of care giver – who should support women during labour?

As previously outlined, continuous support during labour confers a number of benefits. However, although it is well recognised that this approach should be the norm for all women who elect to birth within the hospital setting (Hodnett et al 2007), it is less transparent who is the best person to do so. Consequently, the National Institute for Health and Clinical Excellence (NICE 2007) states that women should be encouraged to have support by birth partners of their choice.

Midwife support

By definition the midwife's role is based on a social and integrated model of care (Walsh and Newburn 2002). This allows for a holistic approach in the assessment, planning, implementation, evaluation, recording, auditing and monitoring of care. Despite the constraints on midwives, they have a wealth of opportunity during their interactions with women and their families to ensure the provision of supportive information through health education/health promotion, and to provide the other dimensions of support outlined earlier in Figure 8.1. But given the different scope to support, it begs the contentious question whether the midwife is the best person to provide all the support the woman needs or can a doula, the woman's partner, female friend or relative play a complementary role, especially during labour? The systematic review by Hodnett et al (2007) suggests that continuous support during labour creates a positive impact when the care giver is not a hospital employee – an interesting finding for midwifery practice. Timing of the onset of continuous support during labour was also evaluated by the researchers as being of significance when it was implemented early. This had beneficial effects in terms of more likelihood of women experiencing spontaneous vaginal births, plus a reduction in need for pharmacological analgesia and caesarean section. The involvement of the midwife in providing informational support to enhance women's coping abilities and to instil confidence is instrumental in the early stages of labour for women labouring at home. Midwives should demonstrate skilled decision-making in order to prevent unnecessary or repeated admissions to hospital, especially for primigravid women (Barnett et al 2008, Cheyne et al 2006, 2007). There should also be scope for midwives to provide support by offering early labour assessment in women's homes (Spiby et al 2006, 2008, Janssen et al 2006).

Doula support

There is a growing body of evidence that the person providing support for women during labour can make a marked difference to outcomes for mother and baby. In terms of support, **doulas** seem to be more beneficial to women psychologically in meeting their emotional needs (Simkin and O'Hara 2002, Hodnett et al 2007, Campbell et al 2006, Scott et al 1999). A doula is a woman who cares for another woman during pregnancy, labour and postpartum. She is not medically trained and does not replace nor compete with the role of the midwife or that of the partner. On the contrary, doulas complement the role of the midwife and partner advocating for women, providing companionship and encouragement as well as informal, practical and emotional support. Women do have to pay for the services of the doula but many find their presence reassuring and comforting in an alien hospital environment.

Partner support

Many women welcome the supportive presence of their partner during labour. However, whilst many women fully embrace the presence and involvement of their baby's father in labour and the birthing process, some have questioned whether men should be present at the birth at all (Chan and Paterson-Brown 2002, Hodnett 2002, Odent 1999) and wonder whether men are fully equipped to guide women through the inherent challenges, pain, stress and anxiety of labour. Odent's (1999) position is that men should not be at the birth as they make the process longer and more difficult as women find it harder to relax; for an explanation why this might be the case see Figure 8.2 and refer to Chapter 6. Now complete the reflective activity in Box 8.3.

Box 8.3 Reflective activity

1. Next time you attend a birth in the home or hospital environment, observe the interactions between the labouring woman and her birth partner.
2. Do you agree with the assertions that men should not be present at birth? Justify your answer.
3. What contribution, if any, can the male partner make in supporting his spouse during labour?
4. How can midwives prepare men who would like to take on a supportive role to their partner during labour?

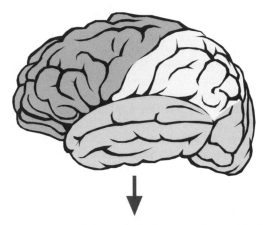

The hormones outlined below are thought to originate in the primitive brain and inhibit neocortical stimulation. However, for this neuro-hormonal response to flow freely the woman needs to feel safe, protected and relaxed. Meaning she must have no worries about how her partner is coping, must not be unduly disturbed and external stimuli such as environmental factors: harsh noise, intrusive language/communication, bright lights and obtrusive observation are counter-productive.

Release of oxytocin, the hormone of love, altruism and social interaction (Odent 1999) is involved in labour, birth, breastfeeding and sexual activity.

Stress response triggers release of catecholamines, produced in response to anxiety and pain.

Production of natural hormonal opiates (beta endorphins) released in presence of painful stimuli but tends to inhibit oxytocin

Equilibrium needs to be established between the flow of the above hormones in order to achieve, maintain and optimise progress in labour.

Figure 8.2 Importance of neuro-hormonal response in labour

Models of good practice

There are many exemplars of good practice that are too many to mention, but there are a few excellent initiatives that justify inclusion.

Albany practice

The Albany Midwifery Practice (AMP) was established in 1997 as a case holding enterprise offering continuity of care to women who are socially disadvantaged in Peckham, an area of South East London, known for its high levels of social deprivation. This was a major public health investment to improve outcomes, including maternal satisfaction, woman-centred care and nurturing, protecting and achieving normality for vulnerable groups of women. The midwives who practise within AMP are self-employed or independent midwives. They operate under contract via King's College NHS Trust, each having their own case load of women (Rosser 2003). The success of this approach to care as reported by Sandall et al (2001) who undertook the initial evaluation of the scheme, has huge ramifications for the organisation and structure of midwifery care in the UK. This is a benchmark model of care that can be replicated nationally if the will and vision is in place. However, in order to fully support women, midwives too need support (Deery and Kirkham 2006). Innovative ways of thinking and working by midwives need support by managers, service providers and the commissioners of maternity care. Lessons can also be learned from the evidence on tried and tested schemes that have a proven track record in reducing morbidity. Case holding offers a real opportunity for midwives to work autonomously and achieve job satisfaction akin to those midwives working in AMP.

One-to-one care in labour

NICE (2007: 73) defines this approach to care as: 'continuous presence and support either by husband/partners, midwives or other birth supporters during labour and childbirth'. The three key recommendations on one-to-one care emerging from this clinical guideline are:

1. Women in established labour should receive care that is supportive via one-to-one care.
2. Women in established labour should not be left alone for long periods.
3. Women should be supported by birth companions of their choice.

Studies such as the one undertaken by Sandall et al (2001), which have evaluated one-to-one midwifery care, consistently demonstrated that women and midwives have a shared vision in striving not only for good outcomes, but also being satisfied with the process of care. Page (2003) states that what pleases women pleases midwives; she argues that just like how women are likely to achieve a sense of personal fulfilment and elation with their birth experience, midwives too get personal job satisfaction by supporting women to realise their birth plan. This serves to build confidence, experience and skills necessary in achieving normality. Table 8.2 illustrates that the notion of continuous support during labour remains an illusory concept for many, despite efforts to ensure that women receive one-to-one care from a midwife when they are in established labour. Women having a home birth or midwifery care in a standalone birthing centre are more likely to experience one-to-one care from a named midwife, unlike those who birth in a hospital setting.

Table 8.2 Findings of the Healthcare Commission Report in England (HCC 2008: 37)

58% of women had the option of a home birth.

40% of births were reported as 'normal'.

20% of women received continuity of care from the same midwife throughout labour.

20% of women reported being left alone in labour to the extent that it worried them.

Family–nurse partnership (FNP)

As stated in Chapter 3, the introduction of FNP is a promising area of development that has undergone rigorous examination regarding its efficacy (Olds 2006). It is a government initiative being piloted in a number of areas, where healthcare professionals provide intensive home visiting for young teenagers who are about to become first time parents and have identified psychosocial factors that make them vulnerable. Nurses or midwives work with first time parents from early pregnancy until the child is 2 years old. Olds (2006) states that FNPs have three main goals, these are:

- to improve pregnancy outcomes by supporting and guiding young mothers and fathers to adopt healthier lifestyles and health behaviours, not only for themselves but also to examine the benefits for their child
- to improve child health and development by good parenting skills and care that is loving and nurturing where the child feels safe and has good role models
- to improve life chances.

Listening visits

Wiggins et al's (2004) study on social support interventions provided postnatally in the form of 'listening visits' by specialist community nurses (health visitors), found that outcomes such as depression and health abusive behaviours, e.g. smoking, were not altered by the intervention but mothers felt more confident in their mothering abilities. Chapter 9 also alludes to the notion of listening visits.

Sure Start

This is an initiative to provide psychosocial support, introduced in 1999 by the UK Government aiming to meet the needs of families with children 0–4 years old, who reside in areas of high socio-economic deprivation (Department of Education and Skills [DES] 2003). The key aim of the scheme is to protect and sure up the health of the nation through providing the next generation with the best possible start in life, achieved via:

- supporting parents in their role as parents and help to meet their aspirations towards employment in order to boost their self-esteem, self-confidence, promote self-efficacy and need for self-determination, and ensuring social cohesion
- increasing the availability of childcare facilities such as children's centres, for all children
- improving the social, physical, psychological, emotional health and cognitive development of children.

Pampering groups

Perry and Alexander's (2006) evaluation of the Sure Start pampering group in Widnes, Chester, provides a clear rationale for such supportive intervention where parents can gather and have 'chill and chat' sessions. They report that the milieu created is one of relaxation where parents feel safe and able to support each other both emotionally and practically, and make decisions in a non-judgemental way. Such pioneering efforts provide opportunities for expectant parents and new parents to network informally and socially. The impetus is to enhance parenting skills, breastfeeding rates through 'buddying' or 'befriending' initiatives, and promote lifestyle changes e.g. less binge drinking, misuse of illicit drugs and strategies to help with the reduction and cessation of smoking in order to achieve better health outcomes.

Role of the midwife

The midwife is charged with the task of supporting women and their partners in order to promote confident parenting skills and emotional wellbeing that will ensure secure attachment relationships with their baby (DH 2004). Providing support also requires the midwife to have skills of collaboration. This is an important function of the midwife's role and a prerequisite to engaging and working with other agencies and members of the multiprofessional team. The midwife also has a role to communicate effectively with women and their families regardless of their background. This includes the skills of active listening and an ability to convey empathetic understanding when supporting families who are vulnerable, disadvantaged or disenfranchised. Psychosocial support is a major determinant of health, helping to combat stress, anxiety and unhealthy lifestyles or abusive behaviour patterns (Wilkinson and Marmot 2003). Sources of stress, anxiety and despair can emanate where there are high levels of social deprivation, mental illness, domestic abuse, lone parenting or bereavement. These factors can take their toll on the individual and can have profound consequences for emotional and psychological health and wellbeing where psychosocial support is lacking.

The very young teenager living in poverty or families more generally who experience high levels of social deprivation are more likely to be uneducated, and struggle financially and emotionally (DH 2004, DES 2003). These families need structured support from the midwife as they reflect the circumstances that make parenting more challenging than usual (D'Souza and Garcia 2004, Vimpani 2000). It is these families that are more likely to exhibit stress and depression and are less skilled to provide the optimum environment that is stimulating and nurturing to child development (Perry and Alexander 2006). It is worth remembering that many of these parents would not have had good parental role models when they too were children.

The midwife providing opportunities for social networking and friendships to develop and flourish will contribute to real change for the families most in need of psychosocial support. Perry and Alexander (2006) have shown that support groups are instrumental in helping to reduce social isolation, boosting confidence and self-esteem, achieving a sense of self-efficacy and supporting women to develop the confidence to breastfeed for as long as possible. Many midwives now work in Sure Start schemes and can make best use of multi-agency working, and ensuring structured antenatal care, continuous support in labour as borne out by the AMP, as well as postnatal visiting planned to meet individual needs. MacArthur et al (2002) noted the marked improvements in the mental health of women who had an increase in midwifery led care from one month to three months postpartum. The involvement of additional community support worker does not appear to have the same effect (Morrell et al 2002). However, the DH (2004) states the need to have a more creative approach to care in the postpartum period – a time of profound adjustment and change (see Chapter 3). Midwives can now extend their visiting up to 90 days, with families most in need of continuity of care (DH 2004). However, there needs to be a major shift in resources, the structure and organisation of care and con-tinued support for midwives within the NHS to make this a reality.

Conclusion

There is clear evidence that support during pregnancy, labour and postpartum is a positive intervention and a major determinant of health for women and their partners as well as assisting parents in meeting the developmental needs of their offspring, especially families with known vulnerability factors. It is clear that the midwife benefits from working in partnership with others in supporting women and meeting their informational, emotional, physical and advocacy needs. The evidence about continuous support in labour is strong and women's perception of support is important. Green et al (2000) has suggested being provided with support and being satisfied with it are two entirely different entities. Social support theory implies that there are positive gains to be had when women perceive that they have readily reliable means of support. In labour the supportive role can be shared by midwives, doulas and a female friend/relative or the partner if that is what the woman wants. The woman's choice of birth companion should always be respected as it is essential that women have an enhanced sense of wellbeing, self-esteem, self-confidence and ability to cope with life transitions or challenges. Midwives practise in a reflective way and increasingly their practice has become grounded in research. This requires midwives to be well informed and to engage with the evidence base to help students they mentor to develop a clear understanding of the different dimensions of support, and the important role support plays in ensuring effective care during the childbearing continuum.

Summary of key points

- Support in pregnancy, labour and postpartum is critical to women's sense of wellbeing helping to promote confident parenting skills and emotional health (DH 2004).

- A high level of psychosocial support especially when provided by significant others such as partner, family members and friends is beneficial to both parenting and child development/behaviour (D'Souza and Garcia 2004, Oakley et al 1996).

- Support is a factor associated with women's satisfaction with the care they received throughout pregnancy and childbirth.

- Structured postnatal visiting, especially for vulnerable groups of women, that allows for increased midwifery care from one month to three months postpartum appear to improve maternal mental health (MacArthur et al 2002).

- The psychosocial dimensions of support prepare parents to effectively engage in healthy parent–infant relationship (Oakley et al 1996). One-to-one care in labour has huge psychological benefits including a positive experience of pregnancy, labour and birth, heightened confidence in parenting skills, and positive emotional well-being. These are just as important as some of the physical outcomes reported such as:

  - reducing likelihood of medical interventions e.g. LSCS
  - reducing need for pharmacological means of analgesia
  - reduction in episiotomy (Hodnett et al 2007, Sandall et al 2001).

References

Barnett, C., Hundley, V., Cheyne, H. and Kane, F (2008) 'Not in labour': impact of sending women home in the latent phase. *British Journal of Midwifery*, 16(3): 144–53.

Campbell, D.A., Lake, M.F., Falk, M. and Backstrand, J.R. (2006) A randomized controlled trial of continuous support in labor by a lay doula. *Journal of Obstetrics and Gynecological Neonatal Nursing*, 35: 456–64.

Chan, K.K.L. and Paterson-Brown, S. (2002) How do fathers feel after accompanying their partners in labour and delivery? *Journal of Obstetrics and Gynaecology*, 22(1): 11–15.

Cheyne, H., Terry, R., Niven, C., Dowding, D.W., Hundley, V. and McNamee, P. (2007) 'Should I come in now?': A study of women's early labour experiences. *British Journal of Midwifery*, 15(10): 604–9.

Cheyne, H., Dowding, D.W. and Hundley, V. (2006) Making the diagnosis of labour: midwives' diagnostic judgement and management decisions. *Journal of Advanced Nursing*, 53(6): 625–35.

Deery, R. and Kirkham, M. (2006) Supporting midwives to support women. In: L.A. Page, R. McCandlish (2006) *The New Midwifery: science and sensitivity in practice*, 2nd edn. Edinburgh: Churchill Livingstone, Chapter 6.

Department of Education and Skills (2003) *Every Child Matters*. London: The Stationery Office.

Department of Health (2008) *Framing the Nursing and Midwifery Contribution: driving up the quality of care*. www.dh.gov.uk, accessed 20 May 2009.

Department of Health (2007) *Maternity Matters: choice, access and continuity of care in a safe service*. www.dh.gov.uk, accessed 20 May 2009.

Department of Health (2004) *National Service Framework for Children, Young People and Maternity Services*. www.dh.gov.uk, accessed 20 May 2009.

D'Souza, L. and Garcia, J. (2004) Improving services for disadvantaged childbearing women. *Child: Care, Health and Development*, 30: 599–611.

Green, J.M., Renfrew, M.J. and Curtis, P.A. (2000) Continuity of carer: what matters to women? A review of the evidence. *Midwifery*, 16(3): 186–96.

Healthcare Commission (2008) *Towards Better Births: a review of maternity services in England*. http://www.cqc.org.uk, accessed 12 June 2009.

Hodnett, E.D. (2002) Pain and women's satisfaction with the experience of childbirth: a systematic review. *American Journal of Obstetrics and Gynecology*, 186(5): S160–S172.

Hodnett, E.D., Gates, S., Hofmeyr, G.J. and Sakala, C. (2007) Continuous support for women during childbirth (Review). *Cochrane Database of Systematic Reviews*, Issue 3. Art No.: CD003766.DOI:10.1002/14651858.

Homer, C., Davis, G., Brodie, P. et al (2001) Collaboration in maternity care: a randomised controlled trial comparing community based continuity of care with standard hospital care. *British Journal of Obstetrics and Gynaecology*, 108: 16–22.

Hunter, B. and Deery, R. (2009) (eds) *Emotions in Midwifery and Reproduction*. Basingstoke: Macmillan.

International Confederation of Midwives (2005) *Definition of the Midwife*. The Hague: ICM.

Janssen, P.A., Still, D.K., Klein, M.C. et al (2006) Early labour assessment and support at home versus telephone triage: a randomized controlled trial. *Obstetrics and Gynecology*, 108(6): 1463–9.

Lewis, G. (ed.) (2007) *Saving Mothers' Lives: reviewing maternal deaths to make motherhood safer 2003–2005. The seventh report on Confidential Enquiries into Maternal Deaths in the United Kingdom*. London: CEMACH.

MacArthur, C., Winter, H.R., Bick, D.E. et al (2002) Effects of redesigned community postnatal care on women's health 4 months after birth: a cluster randomised controlled trial. *Lancet*, 359: 378–85.

McCourt, C., Page, L., Hewison, J. and Vail, A. (1998) Evaluation of one-to-one midwifery: women's responses to care. *Birth*, 25: 73–80.

Martis, R. (2007) *Continuous Support for Women During Childbirth: RHL commentary*. Geneva: World Health Organization. www.who.int, accessed 15 February 2009.

Morrell, C.J., Spiby, H., Stewart, P., Walters, S. and Morgan, A. (2002) Costs and effectiveness of community postnatal workers: a randomised controlled trial. *British Medical Journal*, 321: 593–8.

Murray, E., Keirse, M.J.N.C., Neilson, J. et al (2000) *A Guide to Effective Care in Pregnancy and Childbirth*, 3rd edn. Oxford: Oxford University Press.

National Institute for Health and Clinical Excellence (2007) *Intrapartum Care: care of healthy women and their babies during childbirth*. CG55: London: NICE.

Nursing and Midwifery Council (2004) *Midwives Rules and Standards*. London: NMC.

Oakley, A., Hickey, D., Rajan, L. and Rigby, A. (1996) Social support in pregnancy – does it have long term effects? *Journal of Reproduction and Infant Psychology*, 14: 7–22.

Odent, M. (1999) *The Scientification of Love*, revised edition. London: Free Association Press.

Olds, D.L. (2006) The nurse–family partnership: an evidence-based preventive intervention. *Infant Mental Health Journal*, 27(1): 5–25.

Page, L. (2003) *One-to-one Midwifery Care: restoring the 'with woman' relationship in midwifery*. www.medscape.com, accessed 18 May 2009.

Perry, C. and Alexander, D. (2006) *An Evaluation of the Sure Start Widnes Trailblazer Pampering Group*. Chester: Chester University. www.chester.ac.uk/cphr/reports/036.pdf, accessed 1 June 2009.

Rosser, J. (2003) How do the Albany midwives do it? *MIDIRS Midwifery Digest*, 13(2): 251–7.

Sandall, J., Davies, J. and Warwick, C. (2001) *Evaluation of the Albany Midwifery Practice: Final Report*. London: Florence Nightingale School of Nursing and Midwifery, Kings College.

Scott, K.D., Berowitz, G. and Klaus, M. (1999) A comparison of intermittent and continuous support during labor: a meta-analysis. *American Journal of Obstetrics and Gynecology*, 180(5): 1054–9.

Simkin, P. and O'Hara, M. (2002) Non-pharmacological relief of pain during labour: systematic review of five methods. *American Journal of Obstetrics and Gynecology*, 186: S131–S159.

Spiby, H., Green, J.M., Renfrew, M.J. et al (2008) *Improving Care at the Primary/Secondary Interface: a trial of community-based support in early labour*. The ELSA trial: final report submitted to the National Co-ordinating Centre for NIHR Service Delivery and Organisation (NCCSDO), under peer review. www.sdo.nihr.ac.uk, accessed 1 June 2009.

Spiby, H., Green, J.M., Hucknall, C., Richardson-Foster, H. and Andrews, A. (2006) *Labouring to Better Effect: studies of services for women in early labour*. The OPAL study (Options for Assessment in Early Labour). Report for the National Co-ordinating Centre for NHS Service Delivery and Organisation Research and development. (NCCSDO). www.sdo.nihr.ac.uk/files/project/64-final-report.pdf, accessed 1 June 2009.

Vimpani, G. (2000) Child development and the civil society: does social capital matter? *Journal of Developmental and Behavioural Paediatrics*, 21(1): 44–7.

Walsh, D. and Newburn, M. (2002) Towards a social model of childbirth: Part one. *British Journal of Midwifery*, 10(8): 476–81.

Wiggins, M., Oakley, A., Roberts, I. et al (2004) The social support and family health study: a randomised controlled trial and economic evaluation of two alternative forms of postnatal support for mothers living in disadvantaged inner city areas. *Health Technology Assessment Monograph*, 8(32): 1–134.

Wilkinson, R. and Marmot, M. (eds) (2003) *Social Determinants of Health: the solid facts*. Geneva: World Health Organization (Chapter 7). Available on-line at: www.euro.who.int.

World Health Organization (1999) *Care in Normal Birth: a practical guide*. Geneva: WHO. http://www.who.int, accessed 10 April 2009.

Annotated further reading

Campbell, D., Lake, M., Falk, M. and Backstrand, J. (2006) A randomized control trial of continuous support in labour by a lay doula. *Journal of Obstetrics, Gynecology and Neonatal Nursing*, 34(4): 456–63.

An informative study.

Royal College of Midwives (2008) *Refocusing the Role of the Midwife*. Position Paper, 26. www.rcm.org.uk.

A guidance paper that presents the RCM position on the criteria and fundamental principles that should be used to inform developments aimed at strengthening and refocusing the role of the midwife.

Royal College of Midwives (2004a) *Normal Childbirth*. Position Statement No.4. www.rcm.org.uk.

A useful paper that explores ways to achieve normality in labour and birth.

Royal College of Midwives (2004b) *Doulas*. Position Statement No.6. www.rcm.org.uk.

This paper defines what a doula is and the supportive role provided for women.

Useful websites

Albany Midwives: www.albanymidwives.org.uk
Birth Choice UK: www.birthchoiceuk.com
Fathers direct: www.fathersdirect.com
UK doula support: www.doula.org.uk

9 Attachment and bonding: the midwife's role in supporting parent–baby relationships

Chapter contents

Introduction

Chapter aims

Development of the fetal mind in preparation for emotional interactive relationships

Is the baby primed to attach?

Is the mother primed to make an affectionate bond to her baby?

Meeting their baby for the first time

Mother and baby communication mediated through touch and tenderness

Postnatal activities commonly associated with maternal bonding/relationship building

When separation of parents and baby is needed

Case study: Julie

Case study: Lara

So what can the midwife do?

Conclusion

Summary of key points

References

Annotated further reading

Useful website

Introduction

This chapter will focus upon the issues that surround the creation of relationships that occur in mothers and fathers from birth and beyond, in making meaningful connections with their babies. It will argue that the length of time involved, and what form this relationship takes, is unique to the individuals involved. The Royal College of Obstetricians and Gynaecologists (RCOG 2008) call for the promotion of healthy parent–baby relationships alongside appropriate services and professional interventions that may be required especially where factors exist that are known to inhibit such relationships. The midwife is able to help parents in developing a basic understanding of their role as parent in supporting their baby's mental and emotional development, with an emphasis on effective communication. The view that some people will need specialist input will be explored and recommendations for midwifery practice offered.

Chapter aims

- To examine whether the fetus, baby and mother are biologically and psychologically primed for relationship development

- To explore some of the origins, terminologies, stereotypes and discourses that influence this area of midwifery care

- To suggest that midwives should use clinical guidelines/protocols to provide some standardisation of approach to support mother–baby relationship building in midwifery practice
- To reflect upon current issues related to skin-to-skin contact, breastfeeding and imposed separation of mother and baby
- To offer recommendations for midwifery practice to enhance psychological relationship support for parents and their babies

Development of the fetal mind in preparation for emotional interactive relationships

For the fetus and baby, the mother *is* the environment. The fetus is embraced, rocked and supported in the amniotic fluid in preparation to be held and rocked in her arms in close contact with her body, drinking her colostrum and breast milk, in place of her amniotic fluid. For this sequence of events to happen, Hepper and Shahidullah (1994) believe that the fetus can perceive stimuli and retain some form of memory of it, so that recognition may occur after birth. According to Hepper et al (1993) the mother's voice is perhaps the most salient of all auditory stimuli heard by the fetus which can discriminate after birth between the mother's voice from that of a strange female voice. Hepper et al (1993) suggest that prenatal auditory characteristics of the mother prime the newborn to respond preferentially to its mother and may provide significant feedback to her as she searches for signs of recognition. Thus learning is through exposure and familiarity. Speech development starts immediately after birth and represents a major part of the first social interaction, a process that appears to rely upon the sustained intuitive didactic input of carers. Audition takes centre stage in sensory ability during fetal life so fetal deafness should not be underestimated in its effect on the attachment process. Often the aetiology of deafness is multifactorial and direct links to cognitive brain dysfunction may affect both emotional and general development.

Despite the eye being one of the first organs to be formed, alongside auditory structures, the nature of the intrauterine environment dictates that focus and gaze coordination is developed after birth; however, very shortly after birth, babies are able to recognise their mother's face, and show a preference for the smell and taste of her breast milk (Sparshott 1997). Moreover, Chugani et al (1987) used positron emission tomography to show that fetal limbic and basal ganglion tissues mature in advance of the neo-cortex (see Chapter 7) to enable the baby to engage in expressions of animation and affection. Furthermore, Gerhardt (2004) believes that the orbito-frontal cortex of the brain, part of the pre-frontal cortex and olfactory apparatus (also part of the limbic system) is needed for interpretation of non-verbal cues received from others, which enables the baby to respond in similar style. However, she argues that its development is almost entirely after birth and will depend upon the baby's experience of interaction. With more meaningful interactions, the greater is the growth of this area of the brain. Furthermore, the unique close-fitting tactile stimulation of the uterus provides a special form of touch and proximity that is vital preparation for being held close against the mother's body, being stroked and spoken to in a soft repetitive manner. It appears therefore that the fetus is well prepared for emotional interactive relationships that occur after birth and birth is seen as a transition from one environment to another. Fetal–baby development is part of the same life-span continuum.

Stern (1985) asserts that there are behaviour patterns that are commonly elicited by many people when interacting with babies and are recognised as universal but *sensitive* mothers produce 'supernormal' stimuli. They lean towards their baby, speak in a particularly clear voice, gesture in a slow and deliberate fashion and employ exaggerated facial expressions. Stern's observations show that while the mother steadily provides this consistent intensive stimulation for the baby, the child alternates between attending and not attending. Over time it becomes clear that the patterns of gazing between the two reveal a high degree of synchronisation and reciprocity. The dyadic nature of the sensitivity construct defines it as any pattern of behaviour that pleases the baby, increases the baby's comfort and attentiveness and also reduces distress and disengagement, a pattern that forms the basis for the child's psychological development (Kemppinen et al 2007). The development of baby-to-mother attachment behaviour is a process that extends over many months and years and is the foundation on which toleration of separation as well as exploration of the unfamiliar is in-built (which may appear counter-intuitive; how can attachment mean separation?), but is illustrated in the 'Strange Situation' studies performed by Ainsworth et al (1978) (see Glossary).

Is the baby primed to attach?

While the baby's need for the mother is *absolute*, the mother's need for the baby is *relative*. It is therefore in the baby's interest to activate the mother into close and attentive contact. Babies appear to only offer random confused behaviours, but according to Murray and Andrews (2000) who conducted observational studies, they are highly organised, socially orientated and highly adaptive for survival. Their expressive facial movements and gestures help parents to give them the sensitive care they need. By appreciating the cues they elicit, midwives can help parents become more aware of the richness of their baby's efforts. One of the most dramatic abilities of the newborn is, if content and alert, to gaze intently at the face of another person. If the adult slowly and clearly moves his or her own face, the baby can imitate the other person's facial expression. The baby can show facial expressions such as disgust, sadness, fear and interest. Babies are seen to scan their mother's face taking in each detail, but in turn the mother needs to look at her baby and not all mothers will want or feel able to do this (see Box 9.4).

Attempts at interaction may happen very soon after the birth and the midwife needs to keep environmental interruptions to a minimum during this time. Lighting in the room needs to be relatively low to enable the baby to open his eyes. The baby can similarly interact with his father responding to the sound of his voice. Placed at a distance of 22cm the baby will be able to focus on an object. Sudden noise and bright light will startle the baby and may result in distress (Murray and Andrews 2000), so attempting to partially replicate the conditions of the uterus is a simple guide for midwives to pass on to parents. A soft verbal tone lowers the noise level in the room and loud laughter should always be avoided.

Babies are highly sensitive to their social partner's communication but dislike intrusive social contacts. If the response is too abrupt or before the baby is ready, this may cause a break in engagement. When they begin to tire they yawn, frown, grimace and arch their back. They turn away in an effort to say 'I've had enough'. Some babies cry, others may posset some of their feed. These possets are not associated with feeding but are a need for a reduction in stimulation.

Some babies find being undressed and having their nappy changed distressing. A soft sheet can be used to cover the upper part of the baby to make the baby feel less exposed. Helping the baby to suck upon his fist can help him calm himself if he becomes distressed. A common example is when there is a need for phototherapy using conventional light bank units at the mother's bedside. Placing a baby in contact with the side of the cot and creating confinement with a rolled up sheet may help babies who are initially fretful because of their nakedness and need for more security. This unexpected separation can be stressful for parents and they will both need time to adjust. When the phototherapy lights are switched off for feeding and other care interventions, the midwife should highlight this as vital quality time. It is useful to dim the lighting in the room to enable the baby to re-establish eye contact with his mother. The need for phototherapy is often under-rated by healthcare professionals as a source of anxiety for parents. The midwife's presence and supportive interventions can empower parents to worry less and maintain a positive perception of their baby.

Is the mother primed to make an affectionate bond to her baby?

Bonding

The terms attachment and bonding are often used interchangeably and it appears that, according to Condon et al (2008), as long as the words used convey the intended meaning, practitioners and parents seem not to be too concerned. However, the word bond is applied when the mother feels emotionally connected to her baby. Ainsworth (1991) believes that the word bond should be used as this relationship is not technically an attachment, because a mother does not normally base her comfort and security on her relationship with her baby.

Box 9.1 Bonding: mother–baby togetherness. A legacy of mixed outcomes

Two American paediatricians Klaus and Kennell (1976, 1982) emphasised the mother–baby bond. They highlighted the phenomenon of delight and intimacy manifested by a mother who has an opportunity *immediately post-partum during a critical sensitive period* to hold her baby in close bodily contact and interact with him. They claimed that these mothers displayed better baby care; their children developed better and tended to have fewer later indications of difficulty. Controversially Klaus and Kennell argued that the *critical sensitive period* is when bonding is at its most effective and the mother is hormonally, therefore biologically primed to accept her baby and in its *absence, bonding could not take place*. It was therefore hypothesised that early separation of a newborn and its mother shortly after birth resulted in the mother's possible failure to bond to her baby with lasting consequences for the child as she may neglect or abuse him (Baer and Martinez 2006).

As a direct response to this research, caring for babies in the nursery in the United Kingdom was replaced by *rooming-in*, which meant that the mother cared for her baby at her bedside. She had no choice but to comply. Midwives became teachers of baby care and assessors of whether mothers were, or were not, bonded to their babies. Thus, a more liberating flexibility followed that enabled mothers to engage with their babies from birth.

The researchers were criticised for exaggerating the notion of a *critical sensitive period* that was purely based on animal studies and later acknowledged that they over-emphasised its importance. However, the words had been spoken and written and so became part of the 'consciousness' of the time, indeed their constructions served to impose a new way that mothers *needed* to interact with their baby from birth. Women's magazines and newspapers reported it widely and pregnant women were primed for the new approach. New scripts on how to promote bonding and manage new mothers were written for and by midwives. This new psychological science was influential, but inevitably involved the practice of surveillance and data collection that was used to establish norms for healthy and morally acceptable behaviour against which any person can be assessed.

As a result of the Klaus and Kennell research (see Box 9.1) keeping mother and baby together after birth is considered standard practice, but as Herbert et al (1983) argued then, and is a view that still resonates today, that there are risks of promoting ideas which can become oppressive when they are raised to the status of dogmas. If the notion of engaging in bonding behaviours is imposed and not offered as an opportunity, the mother's choice is denied. When the 'expert' makes the decisions, the mother is left relatively powerless to act. The greatest irony of attachment and bonding discourses is that they destroy what they should seek to defend because the relationship between a mother and her baby is a great intimacy. By applying too much scientific scrutiny to its processes, intimate relationships are rationalised, mothers are judged and judge themselves against the standard of being a 'good enough mother' (Winnicott 1988, 1990). The quality of the bonding process, the amount of time given to it and the anxiety associated with outcome of their child, has resulted in a great deal of unnecessary bad feeling and guilt. Mothers fear being labelled a poor mother. See Box 9.2.

Box 9.2 Reflective activity

1. Is there an unspoken influence in society that makes women feel they should be caring for their baby themselves?
2. Does a maternal instinct exist?

Meeting their baby for the first time

Raphael-Leff (2005) in supporting the psychoanalytic approach, believes that the mother on seeing her baby for the first time has to match it with the imaginary baby that has been growing inside her. This demands an effort of integration that is by no means spontaneous and when the baby is so different from the expected; maternal feelings can range from repulsion to indifference and far from being joyful she may feel cheated as her baby's features are disappointing and so unlike those of her fantasies that she has nurtured for so long. Some women are enraptured by their baby, while others are so exhausted they can only muster enough energy to take a socially acceptable passing interest before handing him over to the father or midwife. A woman exhausted by a perceived long and difficult labour may not want to look at or hold her baby. Indeed how easy is it for a mother to say 'I can't be bothered with him at present' for fear of criticism? It is perhaps the expected thing to give a little lecture on the importance of relationship building, but the midwife who knows that such an intervention is usually counterproductive can demonstrate a non-judgemental attitude and empathy (see Chapter 5) to allay the mother's fears and assure her that her response is both honest and understandable with nothing being lost or undone. Contact with her baby should be determined by the mother's needs (Department of Health (DH) 2007).

In situations when the baby is very different to that expected, for example different sex, gestational age (Niven et al 1993), or the presence of an abnormality (Muggli et al 2009), the mother will need extra continuity and support in the postnatal period which may translate into her being mothered herself. The midwife who can offer a strong model of motherliness may be able to provide some mothers with a guide to mothering behaviour that they may have lacked in the way they were themselves mothered. The midwife does not have to be a biological mother to do this (or female) but offer a level of nurturance, kindness and attention that will help the new mother overcome her grief and/or fear of how to care for her baby by offering encouraging feedback on her strengths and potential (Raphael-Leff 2005).

Social constructions based on maternal instinct see it as a physical attribute that enables the mother to instantly fall in love with her baby: thus some women still believe it a must for bonding to take place for it is the means that enables her to have the *natural* ability to breastfeed and care for her baby with minimal prior instruction or knowledge. Society shapes women's expectations of themselves and for those women who do not get this feeling of overwhelming love immediately they see their baby, may feel something is missing. The less appealing idea of having to 'learn as one goes' can be quite daunting in the reality of caring for a demanding baby and their sense of responsibility to the child can lead to considerable distress in the first few days and weeks of motherhood. Hospital life imposes an interruption from her usual way of coping, separating her from familiar tasks and her support network, which may include neighbours, friends and caring relatives. Learning new skills in a strange situation is more likely to deskill her unless the midwife is seen as a consistently compassionate, patient and good teacher. Place of birth is influential in how women may relate to the people around them (see Chapter 6). Fathers make their own unique contribution to the care and development of the baby; but it is often constructed as different and a later phenomenon (Condon et al 2008).

From a bio-psychological perspective, Swain et al (2007) have reviewed maternal brain blood circuitry using functional magnetic resonance imaging (fMRI) to support a view that the hypothalamic-midbrain-limbic circuits act in concert to support aspects of parental responses to babies, including emotion, attention, motivation, empathy, decision-making and other thinking that are required to navigate the complexities of parenting. Thus the human brain is thought to be 'wired by evolution', to handle a range of social behaviours which overlap with the intense addiction-like concern and focused attention on a preferred individual, similar to the behaviours seen when people fall in love.

Winnicott (1988) coined the words 'primary maternal preoccupations' that constitute almost an illness in their addiction-like aspects of love, obsessions and hyper-vigilance for one's baby. In effect the mother assumes the vulnerability of the baby. He argues that mothers (or mother substitutes) seem to be able to reach this state and it may help them if they can be told by the midwife that these intense feelings will only last a period of time and that they will 'recover' from them, as if they were suffering some form of affliction. He further maintains that many women conceive this state as vegetable-like and in their attempts to counteract its effect, hold on to the very last vestiges of their former life and never surrender to total involvement. Thus these systems seem to be sensitive to a series of important environmental and sensory stimuli that shape their expression and when the parent-baby bond is disrupted, malfunction of these brain circuits can result in anxiety, excessive worrying and obsessive-compulsive disorder (OCD).

Swain et al (2007) argue that mother–baby separation, as a result of extreme prematurity or the presence of major birth defects can deregulate normal motivational feedback mechanisms. Insel (2003) believes that these feedback mechanisms are based on pleasure, baby cries and facial expressions and activate similar brain reward regions that respond when stimulated by cocaine. Thus in non-cocaine addicted mothers, exposure to baby cues appears to be highly reinforcing or at least they invoke motivation to respond. Artificial stimulants such as cocaine may act as a highly reinforcing baby substitute. Confounding influences may include the mother's own adverse childhood experience (which may in turn predispose her to substance abuse). Swain et al (2007) warn that mothers associated with substance abuse and/or clinical depression may abuse or neglect their babies. They argue that maternal behaviours are influenced by current baby cues that activate certain interacting neurotransmitters including oxytocin, prolactin, vasopressin and dopamine.

According to Torner (2008) oxytocin receptors are enriched in brain areas that are significant in the manifestation of social and maternal behaviour including social reduction in stress. Indeed, oxytocin released in mothers during breastfeeding is associated with reduced levels of maternal anxiety and may play a role in rendering the mother more receptive to the trans-mission of baby cues to the mother and encouraging other parenting behaviours. This notion is consistent with the observation that the stress of prolonged mother–baby separation is associated with reduced maternal sensitivity and more negative patterns of mothering (see Case study: Julie).

Swain et al in 2008 used fMRI to show that stimuli produced by the baby activates brain circuitry in the mother that processes motivation, attention and empathy. Among key factors that influence these brain circuits, they consider that the mode of delivery/birth is important in the development of maternal behaviours. The mother's experience of vaginal birth compared with caesarean section (CS) uniquely involves the pulsatory release of oxytocin from the posterior lobe of the pituitary gland. The investigators hypothesised that maternal brain responses to the cries of their own baby at 2–4 weeks postpartum will be enhanced in mothers who have had vaginal births (VB) compared to CS mothers. Related to animal studies, they expected more oxytocin-specific brain activity in the mothers who experienced VB and its associated vaginal-cervical stimulation, compared with CS mothers who were deprived of this physiology. In their small sample of 12 right-handed mothers, 6 had VB and 6 had CS. The researchers assessed their brain activity by comparing their own baby-cry to other baby-cry responses. The fMRI scans showed that the brains of VB mothers, activated areas of the brain known to be associated with certain activities more than the CS mothers. Activations of limbic system structures correlate with abilities for processing vocal emotions and integrating limbic regulation of emotions, an area associated with positive self-conscious emotions, which increases a sense of self-confidence. They found that attending to *own* baby-cry, evoked responses in the brain associated with decision-making in attempting to identify their own baby. Auditory processing and social cognition demonstrated attempts to understand the baby's mental state, leading to more accurate predictions of his/her likely behaviours and needs. This would assist mothers in carrying out appropriate caring behaviours and perform critical interpersonal tasks. It was postulated that perhaps empathic circuits also allow parents to appreciate the discomfort of their baby indicated by their cry.

Evidence of postpartum parental preoccupations was also seen and supports the notion that the same brain circuits that are involved in obsessions and compulsions in regions of the basal ganglia may be activated in postpartum mothers (Mayes et al 2005). On hearing her own baby-cry, this activates regions that normally process face recognition and the researchers think that perhaps the mothers were visualising their baby as they heard their own baby cry. Across the entire sample of own-baby crying a correlation to parental worry, repetitive anxious thoughts and behaviours was found. This may reflect normal and even healthy aspects of adjusting to the new role of mother with associated stress, sleep deprivation and fatigue. To offer this type of information to parents in pregnancy may better prepare them for and create a departure from, the romanticised constructions of new parenthood.

The only area that was more responsive to own baby-cry in CS compared to VB mothers was a region of the brain that processes pain and discomfort. Perhaps there should be more focus on CS mothers and a greater appreciation that their levels of discomfort may be deleterious enough to affect their initial abilities to relate to their babies, which may affect some mothers for weeks after the birth. The factors that surround the need for the caesarean section birth may influence the mother's ability to initially connect with her baby. The process especially if related to an emergency situation may create a psychological separation that is as real as if the baby had been physically taken away. There is general acknowledgement that CS mothers are slower to recover physically, but there is also the cultural expectation of midwives (who are appropriately concerned about the dangers of a surgical birth) that because they are relatively young mothers and not ill, they will jump out of bed and eat a hearty breakfast on the day after surgery. Attempting to care for their baby and recuperate from major surgery can be an ongoing stressful event for many mothers. In such cases, Fieldman (2004) argues for healthcare professionals to empathically encourage the mother–baby relationship but to first ensure that the mother is physically comfortable and pain-free. When procedures are commonplace, the refinements of psychology can get lost in the routines of the day. When everyone around her is seemingly coping, it is difficult for a struggling mother to ask for help. The relationship she desires with her baby may appear as an unachievable distant dream. This notion is supported by Barnes et al (2007) who report that women who had a CS or who have had their babies in the special care baby unit (SCBU) for any time period were more likely to offer negative emotional expressions about them. Their comments were focused to their perceptions of a long-term emotional trauma when the birth did not go smoothly or as planned. The researchers assert that the mother's own health difficulties colour her thoughts and feelings about her baby. With the increase in the CS rate, possibly these mothers are not able to talk to the midwife in sufficient detail about the implications for themselves and their relationship with their baby.

It is tempting to generalise these findings to the wider population and say that VB enhances baby relationship formation in new mothers. However, this cognitive neurobiological approach to psychology in the understanding of affectionate bond behaviour is relatively new and much of the evidence has had to begin with animal studies. It offers a more scientific feel but the psychosocial determinants that can be interpreted from scanning both the parental (and child's) brain) for specific activity, is still speculative. Swain and Lorberbaum (2008) forecast that in the near future, it is hoped that differences in parental response patterns will be reported in specific populations such as those who have securely attached babies, those with postnatal depression and those mothers with a history of substance abuse. This may lead to future assessments of parental mental health risk and resilience profiles using standardised imaging techniques to prevent and treat mental illness that interferes with parenting.

Mother and baby communication mediated through touch and tenderness

In stating the obvious, Winnicott (1988) reinforces the importance of body language. The baby has no verbal language. The willingness and gentleness of being held contributes to a reliable trustworthy feeling for the baby. The mother has been a baby herself. She may have regressed to baby-ways herself during illnesses and possibly formed her own ideas about appropriate baby management. The baby has never been a mother. The baby has not been a baby before. The mother can shrink to infantile modes of experience, but the baby cannot rise to adult sophistication. They learn through exposure to their caregivers. The midwife's role is to help parents to realise that both the mother and baby are continually adapting for a meaningful interaction. If communicated well, this could help parents feel more informed and in control of their new emerging situation. It is inevitable that some babies may be difficult to read; some take longer than expected to respond, some may be over-sensitive and some may react in the only way they know how, by crying. Parents can feel anxious, angry and hopeless in their efforts to understand their baby. The midwife can reiterate these points to parents and may need to point out to them when their baby is signalling for interaction and when he is stressed and needs his own space. Body language is continuously communicated by babies but is often ignored by adults.

It is argued by Ainsworth (1991) (see glossary) that *sensitive* care giving is the key to successful relationship building. The extent to which mothers respond promptly, consistently and appropriately to their baby and hold them carefully with tenderness is said to contribute to a more **secure attachment**. It is further argued that **insecurely attached** babies tend to have mothers who engage in less physical contact, handle them roughly or awkwardly, behave in a routine manner and are sometimes negative, resentful, even rejecting. **Avoidant** babies tend to receive over-stimulating, intrusive care. The mother may talk energetically to them while they are looking away or falling asleep. By avoiding the mother these babies try to escape from overwhelming interaction. **Resistant** babies often experience inconsistent care because their mothers are often unresponsive to their signals.

Postnatal activities commonly associated with maternal bonding/ relationship building

Skin-to-skin contact

The conceptual framework of skin-to-skin contact was first introduced by Klaus and Kennell (1976), particularly for preterm babies that were separated from their mothers. It gradually fell out of favour but was reintroduced during the 1980s into neonatal units such as Kangaroo care (England 2009). The Baby Friendly Initiative (BFI) launched in 1991 (WHO/UNICEF 1989) saw it as a way to place the baby in the vicinity of the breast. After discussion with the mother to inform her of the advantages of skin-to-skin contact, the baby once thoroughly dried is placed onto the mother's naked dry chest. It is argued that such an opportunity should not be denied to any mother, but it is the fine dividing line between a gentle suggestion and an absolute must. The impact of persuasive communications (see Chapter 5) can work to enhance or diminish self-esteem and given that skin-to-skin contact for the first hour of life is used primarily to aid breastfeeding, it is questioned whether the midwife should also refer to relationship building. See Box 9.3.

Box 9.3 Reflective activity

1. Should the activity of skin-to-skin contact be allied to relationship building?
2. To what degree do you refer to relationship building when a mother is formula feeding?

Maternal bonding is generally perceived as one of the advantages of breastfeeding. By pairing these two concepts, if the mother should decide not to have skin-to-skin contact with her baby at all or for less of the recommended time, she may question whether her decision will have a detrimental effect on her relationship with her baby. This framework could be unwittingly supporting the notion of a 'critical sensitive period' (Box 9.1) especially if a timeframe is strictly adhered to. Skin-to skin contact should be encouraged as an ongoing postnatal activity not just confined to the first hour after birth. Many midwives use skin-to-skin contact to enhance neonatal thermo-regulation and it is recommended particularly for the low birth weight baby. With this reasoning in mind, it is argued that the midwife should ensure that all mothers irrespective of their choice of feeding should be given opportunity and encouragement to have skin-to-skin contact with her baby simply because togetherness in touch is a rewarding experience (McKenna and Gettler 2007). The midwife can reassure the parents that the building of relationships between mother and baby, father and baby takes place over a period of time that is not solely dependent upon events that occur immediately around birth.

Breastfeeding

There are many tools in the relationship building kit; breastfeeding is but one and is an extra-ordinarily powerful one. In Western society, many women never hold a newborn baby until they give birth to their own, yet the required frequency of breastfeeding soon makes up for a complete lack of familiarity with babies. According to McKenna and Gettler (2007), the mother and baby are brought into physical and emotional closeness between 8 and 18 times in every 24 hours and she is more likely to rock, speak to and sleep with her baby. There is an assumption therefore that breastfeeding mothers are more emotionally connected to their babies than formula-feeding mothers, but according to Wilkinson and Scherl (2006) there is little empirical evidence to support this view.

These researchers examined the effect of the psychological health of feeding mothers and their attachment styles. Adult attachment styles are the way the person attached to their own mother/caregiver and is said to influence how the person adapts to stress in their daily lives. Secure attachment functions as an inner resource or buffer against stress and allows the person to positively appraise stressful events and turn to others for support and comfort. Insecure attachment styles are either avoidance, ambivalent or dismissing styles and are thought to lead to poor coping.

When applied to childbearing, Mikulincer and Florian (1998) found that securely attached women were found to appraise the task of being a new mother in less threatening terms than avoidant and anxious-ambivalent women. Mothers in both groups were more likely to be feeding their baby as they were fed as a baby. The results showed that breast and formula-feeding mothers did not differ on measures of psychological wellbeing, distress or maternal bonding. They did find however that breast-feeding mothers reported significantly higher levels of secure attachment than formula-fed mothers although there was no significant difference between the groups with regards to insecure attachment styles. It is argued that a secure attachment style helps mothers adjust to possible stresses associated with breastfeeding and to persist with breastfeeding, while insecurity in attachment may hinder such adjustment.

Difficulties in acquiring exclusively formula-feeding mothers for the research skewed the results somewhat as the stigma associated with 'choice of feeding' renders women reluctant to be involved for fear of criticism. The study challenges widely held assumptions about the superior benefits of breastfeeding for the mother and includes the mother's own attachment style as a factor for psychological health which may be helpful to the midwife who is caring for the mother who is struggling to decide whether to continue to breastfeed. By enabling the mother to talk through her reasons for her current indecision/confusion the non-judgemental midwife can give continued support to her and her partner in their choice of feeding, *especially* if she decides to formula feed. For the mother, a feeling of failure and a rejecting attitude from the midwife are not good omens for positive relationship building with her baby (DH 2007).

When separation of parents and baby is needed

Babies that need to be cared for in a neonatal intensive care unit (NICU) are often taken from the birthing room before any skin-to-skin contact is achieved, especially when there is a perceived need for life-saving interventions. These parents are left with empty arms and need tailored emotional support from the midwife. The practice of imposing on the father the role of the communication conduit between the NICU staff and mother, is not always appropriate; can be stressful for him and should take into consideration what he wants to do (DH 2007). Remaining with his partner may be a more natural choice, so that they can support each other. The midwife can act as an advocate for them to stay together and then obtain and relay current information, in a simple, jargon-free manner to them both. Their sense of disappointment and loss is based upon their fear, that their future relationship with their baby is an unknown.

Case study: Julie

Julie birthed her first baby Joe at 28 weeks gestation. He was transferred to the NICU immediately after birth. With her husband Ben, she visited the following day and described her feelings as numb. She said she wanted to hold herself emotionally distant from Joe, in an attempt to lessen the loss if he died. She also commented that he didn't look like a real baby; soft and cuddly. As Joe's condition improved and his survival became reasonably assured, Julie, despite her numerous anxieties about his care, began to have a relationship with Joe.

She performed basic care and got to know him more. If he had a bad day, so it was for her. Gradually she anticipated his homecoming. She said she had increased pleasure and confidence in handling him and a stronger feeling of connection to him.

When she took Joe home she missed the support of the hospital and felt unsure and lacking in confidence. She expressed a need for professional reassurance that she and Ben were making appropriate decisions. They were tired, irritable and amazed at how much Joe cried. They interpreted his crying as their inability to know what he wanted and his persistent crying became an indication that he was a demanding person. Julie's overwhelming tiredness and preoccupation with Joe strained her relationship with Ben. However over time when Julie felt that the rewards exceeded her tiredness and anxiety, Joe would smile at her and she felt appreciated and needed in a special way. Social support from other adults was found to be of great value in coping and maintaining a balanced perspective.

Reid et al (2007), Lupton and Fenwick (2001) and McHaffie (1990) report in their studies that certain women are more at risk for problems in developing a healthy relationship with their baby who is nursed in the NICU. Some of the mothers were not able to say that they were not ready to take their baby home and go to some lengths to conceal their feelings. When asked, they reported that they felt no love for their baby, were not confident in handling him, were angry with him as he was the cause of all their troubles; avoided feeding him and felt irritated by his behaviour. They feared censure or advice from staff who were seen as kind but efficient and knowledgeable, which made them feel inadequate but in sharing their feelings, they were helped to cope as it lifted their burden of worry and guilt.

The primary care midwife needs to continue visiting mothers who take their babies home from the NICU. Some mothers may need extra home visits especially if their pregnancy was unplanned, if they live in poor socio-economic conditions and if they are low in mood. Those who hold inappropriate perceptions of their baby need extra psychological support. In many health authorities, midwives do not offer follow up care for such women. The care is often left to the neonatal services. Multi-agency support must offer early intervention when problems are identified given that the mother's mental health and that of her child could be at risk (DH 2004, 2007, Lewis 2007, Wiggins et al 2004).

Case study: Lara

Lara was having her third baby and always laboured quickly. This time she was only in labour for an hour and birthed James with one small push. However, during skin-to-skin contact she noticed he was breathing quickly. The midwife agreed and called the paediatrician. James was transferred to the NICU with a provisional diagnosis of transient tachypnoea of the newborn. Over the next two days Lara's named midwife on the postnatal ward accompanied her to the NICU to provide support and in addition time was spent with her on the ward, listening to her concerns and anxieties. James was returned to her on his third day. Lara's husband and two daughters visited and were a family reunited in relief and joy. Lara was happy to take James home the following day. The disease was classic in its presentation with minimal ambiguity in diagnosis and a rapid turnaround. Lara felt well supported by the midwife and her family.

Some separations are stressful but not always perceived as a crisis. It is difficult to predict how parents will respond to an unexpected separation from their baby. In the 1970s separation and failure to bond were prescribed as one causing the other but in 1991, Ainsworth acknowledged that few believe there is a 'critical sensitive period' for bonding in humans and despite years of research into the area, still little is known about the processes involved in the formation and maintenance of the maternal bond or even of the criteria that marks its establishment. Mothers may be responsive and accessible carers but not all babies become securely attached to their mothers and not all mothers who become bonded to their baby fit suggested criteria. Even mothers who demonstrate less than ideal care of their babies usually do not want them removed from their care; they are possibly bonded to them in their own way.

Box 9.4 Psychosocial factors that may influence the relationship between the mother and her baby. Would your list differ in any way?

Maternal sensitivity and responsiveness

Evidence of post-traumatic stress disorder in either or both parents

Good relationships with own parents

Quality of mother's relationship with the father of the baby

Poverty

Low income household

History of antenatal depressive illness

Ongoing postnatal depressive illness

Ambiguity of outcome of baby's health

Mode of delivery/birth

Separation from baby, initially sick, usually LBW with need for NICU/SCBU

Fussy baby temperament

An 'unsocial' baby

Unwanted pregnancy

History/current substance abuse in either/both parents

The mother's coping style

Lack of enjoyment of feeding

Stress and anxiety in the transition to parenthood

Perception of own attachment experience as a child

Effective or lack of social support

Early intervention when problems arise

Supportive birth experience

Continuity of carer

Homebirth

Very young parents

Bereavement especially with surviving twin

IVF assisted pregnancies.

Supporting references: Baer and Martinez (2006); Barnes et al (2007); Kemppinen et al (2007); Mantymaa et al (2006); Steadman et al (2007).

So what can the midwife do?

- foster mother–baby, father–baby relationships
- acknowledge that relationship building is not necessarily time or event related
- know there are no set criteria on which parents should be judged whether they are bonded/attached to their baby
- create/update guidelines that provide a dialogue that enables them to relay information that is helpful, truthful, challenging to parents; with a sense of 'knowing what to say and how to say it'
- consider factors that may influence the parent–baby relationship (see Box 9.4)
- engage in multi-agency collaboration when referral is deemed necessary.

Conclusion

Attachment and bonding processes remain an important part of a midwife's work. Timely and effectively communicated information about how the baby and parents are able to develop a meaningful relationship should be offered, but it should be emphasised that when (and if) it occurs its nature will be as unique as the individuals involved. Breastfeeding and skin-to-skin contact are associated with relationship building and are desirable but neither is essential for it to happen. The mother who chooses to formula feed is especially vulnerable for she represents the 'non-compliant other', and must not feel any sense of being less. Separation of mothers and babies should always be avoided and sometimes the harsh environment of the birthing room and the need to perform routine tasks create unintentional interruptions to initial 'getting to know you' processes. When separation is as a result of a need for special or intensive care, the midwife can coordinate a link with the team who are caring for the baby and support each parent in how they wish to manage their situation. The relationship with their baby may take a different path given all the variables of having a baby that is sick, but having a meaningful relationship whenever it happens, should be anticipated. The need for written guidelines can be helpful in providing a dialogue/record for midwives to discuss what they say and how they say it and what constitutes a need for referral. Early intervention through continuity of support in primary care should be provided for families at risk with the midwife working as a member of a multi-agency team. Psychological support through listening visits and confidence building can help to safeguard the baby's development and growth.

Summary of key points

- Both mothers and babies are primed for interaction. Midwives can help parents become more informed about these processes to help them feel more in control.

- The baby's survival is based on its ability to stimulate interaction with the mother.

- There is no set time for when parents will form meaningful relationships with their baby. A 'critical sensitive period' when the mother should bond to her baby following birth, is no longer thought valid.

- New bio-psychological methods are adding a fresh dimension to the existing body of research and may help a new mother to understand that her new emerging behaviour patterns are part of an adaptive process to help her cope with her new role.

- Midwives can support parents in relationship building by creating conditions in the birthing room that are free from unnecessary interruptions, with appropriate lighting and noise levels.

- The mother's choice in whether she wishes skin-to-skin contact and how she chooses to feed her baby is hers and no persuasion or coercion should link these concepts with relationship building.

- Comprehensive guidelines should form a standard that is able to inform midwives of parental behaviour that falls outside normal parameters to help them to know when to refer to other agencies.

References

Ainsworth, M.D.S. (1991) Attachments and other affectionate bonds across the life cycle. In: C.M. Parkes, J. Stevenson-Hinde, P. Marris (eds) *Attachment across the Life Cycle*. London: Routledge, pp 140–50.

Ainsworth, M.D.S, Blehar, M., Walters, E. and Wall, S. (1978) *Patterns of Attachment*. Hillsdale, NJ: Erlbaum.

Baer, J.C. and Martinez, C.D. (2006) Child maltreatment and insecure attachment: a meta-analysis. *Journal of Reproductive and Infant Psychology*, 24(3): 187–97.

Barnes, J., Ram, B., Leach, P. et al: The Families, Children and Child Care Project Team (2007) Factors associated with negative emotional expression: a study of mothers of young infants. *Journal of Reproductive and Infant Psychology*, 25(2): 122–38.

Chugani, H.T., Phelps, M.E. and Mazzotta, J.C. (1987) Positron emission tomography study of human brain functional development. *Neurology*, 22: 587–97.

Condon, J.T., Corkindale, C.J. and Boyce, P. (2008) Assessment of postnatal paternal-infant attachment: development of a questionnaire instrument. *Journal of Reproductive and Infant Psychology*, 26(3): 195–210.

Department of Health (2007) *Maternity Matters: choice, access and continuity of care in a safe service*. London: DH.

Department of Health (2004) *National Service Framework for Children, Young People and Maternity Services*. Standard 11. London: DH.

England, C. (2009) The healthy low birthweight baby. In: D. Fraser and M.A. Cooper (eds) *Myles Textbook for Midwives*, 15th edn. London: Churchill Livingstone.

Fieldman, R. (2004) Mother skin-to-skin contact and the development of emotion regulation. *Advances in Psychology Research*, 27: 113–31.

Gerhardt, S. (2004) *Why Love Matters*. Hove: Brunner-Routledge.

Hepper, P.G. and Shahidullah, S. (1994) The beginnings of mind – evidence from the behaviour of the fetus. *Journal of Reproductive and Infant Psychology*, 12(3): 143–54.

Hepper, P.G., Scott, D. and Shahidullah, S. (1993) Newborn and fetal response to maternal voice. *Journal of Reproductive and Infant Psychology*, 11(3): 147–53.

Herbert, M., Slukin, W. and Slukin, A (1983) Mother-to-infant bonding. *Journal of Child Psychology and Psychiatry*, 23(3): 205–21.

Insel, T.R. (2003) Is social attachment an addictive disorder? *Physiology and Behaviour*, 79: 351–7.

Kemppinen, K., Raita-Hasu, J., Toivonen-Falck, A. et al (2007) Early maternal sensitivity and child behaviour at toddler age: does low maternal sensitivity hinder identification of behavioural problems? *Journal of Reproductive and Infant Psychology*, 25(4): 270–84.

Klaus, M.H. and Kennell, J.H. (1982) *Parent–Infant Bonding*. St. Louis: Mosby.

Klaus, M.H. and Kennell, J.H. (1976) *Maternal–Infant Bonding*. St. Louis: Mosby.

Lewis, G. (ed.) (2007) *Saving Mothers' Lives: reviewing maternal deaths to make motherhood safer 2003–2005*. The seventh report on Confidential Enquiries into Maternal Deaths in the United Kingdom. London: CEMACH.

Lupton, D. and Fenwick, J. (2001) 'They've forgotten that I'm the mum'; constructing and practising motherhood in special care nurseries. *Social Science and Medicine*, 53(8): 1011–21.

Mantymaa, M., Tamminen, T., Puura, K., Luoma, I., Koivisto, A. and Salmelin, R. K. (2006) Early mother–infant interaction: associations with the close relationships and mental health of the mother. *Journal of Reproductive and Infant Psychology*. 24, 3, 213–231.

McHaffie, H.E. (1990) Mothers of very low birthweight: how do they adjust? *Journal of Advanced Nursing*, 15: 6–10.

McKenna, J.J. and Gettler, L.T. (2007) Mother–infant co-sleeping with breastfeeding in the western industrialized context. In: T.W. Hale and P.E. Hartmann (eds) *Textbook of Human Lactation*. Texas USA: Hale Publishing, pp 271–302.

Mayes, L.C., Swain, J.E. and Leckman, J.F. (2005) Parental attachment systems: neural circuits, genes, and experiential contributions to parental engagement. *Clinical Neuroscience Research*, 4: 301–13.

Mikulincer, M. and Florian, V. (1998) The relationship between adult attachment styles and emotional cognitive reactions to stressful events. In: J.A. Simpson and W. S. Rholes (eds) *Attachment Theory and Close Relationships*. New York: Guildford Press, pp 200–10.

Muggli, E., Collins, V. and Marraffa, C. (2009) Going down a different road: first support and information needs of families with a baby with Down syndrome. *Medical Journal of Australia*, 190(2): 58–61.

Murray, L. and Andrews, L. (2000) *The Social Baby*. Surrey: CP Publishing.

Niven, C., Wiszniewski, C. and AlRoomi, L. (1993) Attachment (bonding) in mothers of preterm babies. *Journal of Reproductive and Infant Psychology*, 11: 175–85.

Raphael-Leff, J. (2005) *Psychological Processes of Childbearing*. London: The Anna Freud Centre.

Reid, T., Bramwell, R., Booth, N. and Weindling, A.M. (2007) A new stressor scale for parents experiencing neonatal intensive care: the NUPS(Neonatal Unit Parental Stress) scale. *Journal of Reproductive and Infant Psychology*, 25(1): 66–82.

Royal College of Obstetricians and Gynaecologists (2008) *Standards for Maternity Care*. Report of a working party. London: RCOG Press.

Sparshott, M. (1997) *Pain, Distress and the Newborn Baby*. London: Blackwell Science.

Steadman, J., Pawlby, S., Mayers, A., Bucks, R.S., Gregoire, A., Miele-Norton, M. and Hogan, A.M. (2007) An exploratory study of the relationship between mother–infant interaction and maternal cognitive function in mothers with mental illness. *Journal of Reproductive and Infant Psychology*. 25, 4, 255–269.

Stern, A. (1985) *The Interpersonal World of the Infant*. New York: Basic Books.

Swain, J.E. and Lorberbaum, J.P. (2008) Imaging the human parental brain. In: R.S. Bridges (ed.) *Neurobiology of the Parental Brain*. London: Academic Press, Elsevier.

Swain, J.E., Tasgin, E., Mayes, L.C., Feldman, R., Constable, R.T. and Leckman, J.F. (2008) Maternal brain responses to own baby-cry is affected by cesarean section delivery. *Journal of Child Psychology and Psychiatry*, 49(10): 1042–52.

Swain, J.E., Lorberbaum, J.P., Chose, S. and Strathearn, L. (2007) Brain basis of early parent–infant interactions: psychology, physiology and *in vivo* functional neuroimaging studies. *Journal of Child Psychology and Psychiatry*, 48(3): 262–87.

Torner, L. (2008) Role of prolactin in the behavioural and neuroendocrine stress adaptations during lactation. In: R.S. Bridges (ed.) *Neurobiology of the Parental Brain*. London: Academic Press, Elsevier.

Wiggins, M., Oakley, A., Roberts, I. et al (2004) The social support and family health study: a randomised controlled trial and economic evaluation of two alternative forms of postnatal support for mothers living in disadvantaged inner city areas. *Health Technology Assessment Monograph*, 8(32): 1–134.

Wilkinson, R.B. and Scherl, F.B. (2006) Psychological health, maternal attachment and attachment style in breast- and formula-feeding mothers: a preliminary study. *Journal of Reproductive and Infant Psychology*, 24(1): 5–19.

Winnicott, D.W. (1990) *The Maturational Process and the Facilitating Environment*. London: Karnac Books.

Winnicott, D.W. (1988) *Babies and their Mothers*. London: Free Association Books.

World Health Organization/UNICEF (1989) *Joint Statement – Protecting, Promoting and Supporting Breastfeeding*. Geneva: WHO.

Annotated further reading

Bertram, L. (2008) *Supporting Postnatal Women into Motherhood*. Oxford: Radcliffe Publishing.

An insightful read into difficulties experienced and how women may be helped and supported in the postnatal period.

Crittenden, P.M. and Hartl-Claussen, A. (eds) (2003) *The Organisation of Attachment Relationships: maturation, culture and context*. Cambridge: Cambridge University Press.

This text broadens the range of attachment theory by putting forward an alternative view to take account of childbearing practices across cultures.

Useful website

www.baby.friendly.org.uk/health

10 Psychological care matters

Chapter contents

Introduction

Chapter aims

The argument for psychology in midwifery
practice

The psychological impact of caring for
vulnerable women

The importance of the care environment

Future challenges

References

Annotated further reading

Introduction

This concluding chapter will argue that focusing on the psychological aspects of a woman enables the midwife to relate to and understand her behaviour more thoroughly and is a means to meet her needs more effectively. However some midwives only focus on the social and biophysical aspects of care and seem not to recognise the value of psychological health, which affects the mother, her baby and her family. In situations where extra vulnerability exists, it is argued that certain psychological interventions can be supportive, especially where there are perinatal mental health or domestic violence issues that need a sensitive approach. The psychology of stress and anxiety experienced in migrant families will be explored and its effects upon maternal attachment behaviour. The medical label of 'high risk' is examined and how it affects women who are hospitalised, their coping strategies and how they perceive the quality of their attachment to their baby as a result of being labelled thus. 'Being a good mother' is conceptualised as a social construction and relates to how women strive to achieve the best they can be. The care environment shapes and defines behaviour and primary care places the woman in her natural environment and the home, for most women, remains the most fitting psychological setting. Present funding and care strategies will need revising to meet the future demands of social policies that call for qualitative changes to care that truly meet the holistic needs of women. To do this, midwives need to feel cared for too. These needs are emphatically psychological in origin.

Chapter aims

- To give a short rationale that questions why midwives may not engage with psychology to support their practice
- To promote the view that there is a symbiotic relationship between psychology and midwifery practice that needs to be nurtured further

- To offer a reflection of the book chapters by briefly exploring a theme of vulnerability in childbearing women and how the midwife may provide psychological support and guidance

- To reinforce that the care environment is influential in how people behave and the home should always remain a place of choice for those women who desire it

- To acknowledge that midwives do demanding work with many conflicting tensions and how a psychological approach may assist the midwife to find more cohesive ways of managing self

The argument for psychology in midwifery practice

The potential for psychology in midwifery care is unlimited because it informs one's under-standing of human behaviour and endeavour. Psychology is about attempting to open doors, to try to understand what matters to the people who give and receive midwifery and childbearing health care. Midwives need to engage with psychology and integrate it into their thoughts and actions so that it becomes part of their attitudes and behaviour (see Figure 10.1).

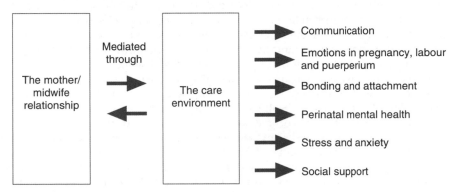

Figure 10.1 The psychological context of midwifery care

It is acknowledged that some midwives are not familiar with psychology and as a result perhaps do not recognise its value. The reasons may be that:

- they have not studied psychology therefore have little knowledge of its structures, com-ponents and relevance to the human mind, spirit and behaviour of a person
- those who have studied psychology experienced a more general approach with little applica-tion to health care
- they have limited knowledge of what aspects of psychology are recognised as applicable and valid in midwifery practice.

Some midwives see psychology as an 'ology' and therefore part of an unnecessary theoretical construct based on ideals that cannot be achieved in practice. They imply they are 'too busy for psychology' which may be interpreted that they only engage with 'touchy-feely' stuff when they have time to do so and then only as 'added extra' to their routine work.

This is not how psychology should be perceived. The focus of this book applies to the daily work of midwives; psychology goes to the core of what midwives do. The relationship she has with the woman and the development of a rapport is vital in the offering and receiving of care (Chapters 2 and 5). Psychology can teach the midwife that the woman may experience a diverse range of emotions before, during and after her baby is born, but also warns that emotional behaviour can be stereotyped by society (see Chapter 3). There are always exceptions to the rule and for those women who are not emotional, or do not wish to show their emotion, they should not be judged as abnormal or deviant. A psychological approach provides a guide to offering care that is truly suited to the woman. It is inclusive to all women in society and respects their dignity and personal integrity which in turn protects and sustains their wellbeing.

Reflective activity

An experienced midwife was heard to say, 'I think I give excellent care . . . I treat all women the same.'

What are your views on the midwife's statement?

This comment implies that the midwife offers an acceptable standard of care and perhaps does not explicitly disadvantage any of the women in her care, but to what extent is her care woman-centred? Are the women's psychosocial health needs being satisfied? Does each individual woman feel that her interaction with the midwife is personally focused upon her and does this raise the woman's self-esteem and sense of self-efficacy? To psychologically empower a mother to feel better about herself (and her situation) means that the midwife is able to make each interaction a qualitatively enriching and fulfilling experience for the woman. The woman is more likely to thrive when treated this way and better able to make her own decisions about the type of care she desires because she is confident to choose from the options available. As depicted in Chapter 2, a relationship of sharing, where the woman takes hold of her own power to be completely self-directed, is a source of affirmation to the midwife. Reciprocity is an important paradigm for midwives. The relationship with women needs to be anchored and centred to ensure trust and cooperation.

Psychology principles are applied to all midwifery situations, but it is particularly useful when the midwife senses that the task before her may threaten her own personal resources. She may question whether she has the skills and experience to cope. Each midwife will have her own notion of what represents a personal threat or challenge, but caring for the most vulnerable women in society is a common ground for concern.

The psychological impact of caring for vulnerable women

Perinatal mental illness, domestic violence, lone parenting and bereavement (see Chapters 4 and 8) are areas that midwives may find particularly difficult. Midwives need to ask themselves whether they are thoroughly prepared, willing and able to talk about issues that may have resonance within their own life or simply find them too personal to mention. They need to question whether they are acting in such a way that creates a communication window to enable the woman to tell her story. The fear of social stigmatisation remains a threat to the woman's safety needs and unless the midwife can relay her positive beliefs and attitudes regarding safe disclosure, the woman may keep her thoughts to herself. The midwife's use of an appropriate facial expression, tone of voice, quietness, even silence may be enough to cue the woman that she is worthy of the time spent with her. If there is the mere suggestion of the midwife hurrying the appointment along, the opportunity may be squandered. Midwives need to be mindful of flexible appointment systems that facilitate and support the telling of the most sensitive stories. The midwife's active listening skills and referral abilities, her sense of timing and symmetry are often pivotal in supporting a woman in great need (see Chapter 1).

Working with the stresses of cultural diversity and its effects on maternal prenatal attachment behaviour

Another area of care that calls for midwife fortitude and strength of character is caring for women where cultural differences may cause unwanted division and awkwardness. Language difficulties may range from not sharing a common language to inappropriate cultural inter- pretations of meaning that words and phrases may inadvertently convey. The process is time-consuming, complex and can be a source of fatigue and frustration for both parties. MacLachlan (2004) asserts that families who have left their own country either as temporary sojourners or permanent migrants, whether forced (involuntary) migrants or refugees, have the stresses and strains of adjustment to deal with. Some are young teenage women; others have poor maternal health that places them in a high-risk category, which may warrant hospitalisa- tion (Lewis 2007). Stress and anxiety is a common feature in the behaviour of such women and the midwife can help in understanding the different causal types of stress and take account of their recent history. Acculturative stress is when people value their heritage culture relative to the one they have migrated into and can seriously affect physiological, psychological and social aspects of health. Integration (wishing to identify with the host culture and the culture of origin) is a more beneficial strategy in terms of maintaining mental health than marginalisation (wishing to identify with neither). Assimilation (identifying only with the host culture) and separation (identifying only with the culture of origin) are associated with intermediate levels of stress. In a cross-cultural study, Bielawska-Batorowicz and Siddiqui (2008) considered whether there are cultural differences in prenatal attachment styles in Swedish and Polish mothers and found that the conceptualisation of the relationship with the unborn baby is similar. Complications of pregnancy might affect the attachment process attributed to dif- ferences in the woman's perception and experience of health care. It is suggested that women who do not feel comfortable in the healthcare system react to pregnancy complications with increased concentration on their own wellbeing and thus withdraw some of their emotions from the relationship with their developing baby. Migration results in many women birthing their babies outside their usual cultural milieu and the woman's social construction of mother- hood could differ considerably, such as her approach to pain and its management. Midwives should be sensitive to different cognitions and attitudes including those to unborn babies that may affect women's health related behaviours in pregnancy, especially if they are stressed and unhappy.

Managing 'high risk' pregnancy stress and its effects on prenatal attachment behaviour

Women can feel particularly vulnerable when their pregnancy is medically deemed as high risk and White et al (2008) found that when women adopted positive appraisal coping strategies (Lazarus and Folkman 1984) they experienced less distress. Their positive appraisal of threat appeared to be important in the development of the prenatal attachment relationships to their baby. The challenge of developing midwife interventions to promote positive appraisal coping strategies for women with complicated pregnancies lies in the sensitive balance between the realistic medical risk in the pregnancy and challenging negative hopeless appraisals that might inhibit attachment behaviours. Midwives need to acknowledge the woman's appraisal of risk and should remain aware of the potential discrepancies between their own opinions and the need to create an environment where there is promotion of the positive aspects of their pregnancy and praising the woman's attempts to cope with difficult circumstances. Above all the woman should feel free to discuss her fears with her named midwife, who makes herself available to her. Anxiety was found to adversely affect maternal appraisals and intensity of attachment in women who were having a pregnancy after a previous perinatal loss. It is not surprising that appraisal of threat to the current pregnancy results in increased anxiety and reduced attachment behaviour (Côté-Arsenault 2007) (see Chapters 7 and 9).

Supporting motherhood

According to Moller et al (2008), the impact of a new baby and the qualitative support of the partner can be influential in how the woman negotiates her psychosocial transition to parenthood, especially if there are co-existing factors that work against the couple like financial impoverishment, disability or poor/absent family social support (see Chapters 3 and 8). Society expects women to be natural, intuitive and instinctive mothers. Brown et al (1997) asked Australian women what they thought constituted 'being a good mother'. The researchers reported how struck they were by the energy and commitment the women gave to motherhood. Most women accepted the impossibility of fulfilling their ideal of being a good mother all of the time, but their accounts nevertheless reflected the strain of trying to live up to it. There remains a heavy burden on women in attempting to reconcile pervasive beliefs about being a good mother with the many competing demands on their physical and psychic energy. The midwife can be instrumental in deconstructing the myths of motherhood and fatherhood to enable parents to minimise the 'oughts and shoulds' of social pressure from well-meaning but influential others.

The importance of the care environment

From a feminist perspective, Bates (2004) argues that the primary care setting positions midwifery practice in its social context and the woman's choice of a home or clinic environment should be made available. The slow but erosive loss of home visit practice is a detrimental step because context dictates how people behave (see Chapter 6) and the woman in her own home offers a great deal of information for the midwife to assess and plan her psychological care. Where mental health vulnerability exists and the woman desires it, regular home visits may enhance her relationship with her baby, her partner and her family. The midwife can offer a life-line of continuity of contact and social support.

Future challenges

Whether in a hospital or primary care setting, the care environment of the future needs to support the woman, her family, the midwife and her team. This includes the student midwife who will learn what she observes (Bandura 1977). It is not psychologically sound for an organisation to set people to work in a system where more is expected of them than what they can possibly deliver. This applies to the number of women midwives are asked to care for at any one time and the level of each woman's vulnerability and neediness. The Department of Health (DH 2003) states that the environment in which care takes place in modern healthcare settings is often highly complex and pressurised. Quality communication is often the first casualty as cognitive appraisal of threat corrupts mental agility, decision-making and concentration. As coping strategies become less effective they are replaced by chronic fatigue and exhaustion, which may become the norm for that person. This way of living eventually leads to disillusionment and failure and is a poor model for the student midwife. This book will hopefully be a source of insight and motivation for midwives and students to create more effective ways to achieve quality, woman-centred care that is grounded in an applied psychological framework. A psychological approach can help midwives to understand their own cognitions and enable them to ask for what they need to practice effectively. Psychology is the study of mind spirit and behaviour and therefore applies to all people and by the same token, all people can benefit from it.

References

Bandura, A. (1977) *Social Learning Theory*. Englewood Cliffs, NJ: Prentice-Hall, pp 58, 91.

Bates, C. (2004) Midwifery practice: ways of working. In: M. Stewart (ed.) *Pregnancy, Birth and Maternity Care. Feminist perspectives*. London: Books for Midwives, pp 121–42.

Bielawska-Batorowicz, E. and Siddiqui, A. (2008) A study of prenatal attachment with Swedish and Polish expectant mothers. *Journal of Reproductive and Infant Psychology*, 36(4): 373–84.

Brown, S., Small, R. and Lumley, J. (1997) Being a 'good mother'. *Journal of Reproductive and Infant Psychology*, 15(2): 185–200.

Côté-Arsenault, D. (2007) Threat, appraisal, coping and emotions across pregnancy subsequent to prenatal loss. *Nursing research*, 56, 108–16.

Department of Health (2003) *Making Amends – a consultation paper setting out proposals for reforming the approach to clinical negligence in the NHS*. www.dh.gov.uk, accessed 22 July 2009.

Lazarus, R.S. and Folkman, S. (1984) *Stress, Appraisal and Coping*. New York: Springer.

Lewis, G. (ed.) (2007) *Saving Mothers Lives: reviewing maternal deaths to make motherhood safer 2003–2005*. The seventh report on Confidential Enquiries into Maternal Deaths in the United Kingdom. London: CEMACH.

MacLachlan, M. (2004) Culture, empowerment and health. In: M. Murray (ed.) *Critical Health Psychology*. London: Palgrave Macmillan, pp 101–17.

Moller, K., Hwang, C.P. and Wickberg, B. (2008) Couple relationship and transition to parenthood: does workload at home matter? *Journal of Reproductive and Infant Psychology*, 26(1): 57–68.

White, O., McCorry, N.K., Scott-Hayes, G., Dempster, M. and Manderson, J. (2008) Maternal appraisals of risk, coping and prenatal attachment among women hospitalised with pregnancy complications. *Journal of Reproductive and Infant Psychology*, 26(2): 74–85.

Annotated further reading

Page, L. and McCandlish, R. (2006) *The New Midwifery*, 2nd edn. Edinburgh: Churchill Livingstone.

A key text for midwifery practice.

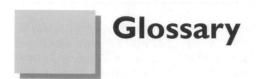

Glossary

Affectional bond   the strong affectionate tie in which the partner is important as a unique individual, interchangeable with none other.

Agoraphobia   an anxiety disorder that is often precipitated by the fear of experiencing a panic attack in an environment from which the sufferer cannot readily escape. Consequently, agoraphobics may avoid public places/public transport.

Anhedonia   lack of the pleasure principle or an inability to experience joy from normally pleasurable events.

Attachment   an affectionate bond and hence an attachment figure is never wholly interchangeable with or replaceable by another, even though there may be others to whom one is attached. What distinguishes attachment from an affectional bond is seeking to obtain an experience of security and comfort in the relationship with the partner. When available the individual is able to move off from the secure base provided by the partner with confidence to engage in other activities. This is the essence of an attachment and the reason why the mother is said to bond to her baby.

Bipolar illness   this condition in the past was commonly referred to as manic-depressive illness. Features of psychosis are apparent (hallucinations and delusions). There is marked cognitive and affective dysfunction that causes major disruptions in the person's mood, energy and ability to function. The symptoms of bipolar disorder are severe with suicide a real threat.

Body image   The mental image of one's body and thoughts as well as feelings.

Body mass index (BMI)   a formula used to calculate and compare a person's weight (in kilograms) divided by the square of his/her height (in metres). This gives a crude population measure on whether the individual is considered underweight, normal weight, overweight, obese or morbidly obese.

Debriefing   a psychological intervention used as a one-off, semi-structured conversation with an individual who has just experienced a stressful or traumatic life event. The main purpose of debriefing is to reduce any possibility of psychological harm by allowing the individual to talk about the traumatic experience to help make sense of what happened.

Delusion   a fixed false belief that is impenetrable to reason.

Discourse   spoken or written words, images, metaphors, that construct an object in a particular way.

Disinhibition   in the field of psychiatry, this relates to losing inhibition and displaying uncharacteristic behaviour. For the childbearing woman, this might involve her stripping off her clothes and acting in a sexually suggestive manner, which increases her vulnerability.

Domestic abuse   the preferred terminology adopted by the Department of Health in England that relates not only to physical violence but any incident of threatening behaviour, abuse or violence be it physical, psychological, emotional, sexual or financial that occurs between adults who are or have been intimate partners or family members, regardless of gender or sexuality.

Doula a paid helper or woman who cares for another woman during pregnancy, labour and puerperium. She is not medically trained and her main role is to offer companionship, practical help and support and where necessary advocate for the woman.

Emotion work work undertaken to manage feelings and achieve congruence between emotions and behaviour.

Fetocide the destruction of a fetus in utero. In the UK selective fetocide might be advised in the case of multiple pregnancy to enhance the chances of realising a live birth for the remaining fetus if twin pregnancy or twins in the case of a triplet pregnancy.

Free birthing where a woman elects to birth her baby without the support, guidance, skilled knowledge and help of a midwife or doctor.

Hallucination a sensory perception in the absence of a stimulus. This can affect any of the five senses, e.g. seeing objects that are not present, hearing imaginary voices, smelling foul/pungent odours, feeling strange sensations (tactile hallucinations) or perceiving strange tastes. Individuals who experience hallucinations believe the perception is real.

Hegemony dominant ideology or dominant leadership of a particular social order/group.

Incidence number of individuals who become ill who have been previously well.

Insecure-ambivalent the infant is distressed and highly focused on the parent, but cannot be settled by the parent on reunion, often expressing anger and seeking contact in quick succession and generally failing to return to play. This category is associated with maternal insensitivity and unpredictability of maternal responsiveness.

Insecure-avoidance the infant shows few or no signs of missing the parent and actively ignores and avoids her on reunion. This pattern is associated with maternal insensitivity to infant signals and specifically with rejection of attachment behaviour.

Insecure-disorganised/disorientated the infant exhibits a diverse array of behaviours such as freezing all movements, wearing a dazed facial expression sometimes expressing a flat depressed emotion. The mothers show characteristics of any of the other categories. At the same time they reason in a disorganised and confused way.

Panopticism a social theory that emerged from the work of the French philosopher Michel Foucault that addresses a broad, comprehensive or microscopic view of issues.

Perinatal psychiatric illness/perinatal mental illness now the accepted term used both nationally and internationally to emphasise the importance of psychiatric disorder in pregnancy as well as following childbirth. It highlights the range of mental illness that can affect women during the childbearing years.

Power is multi-dimensional and literally means to have agency or an ability to influence, respond, bring about or effect change.

Powerlessness rendered helpless, lacking agency, devoid of ability or power to influence, respond or effect change. This often results in an air of resignation where the powerless person feels trapped, stuck in a rut, hopeless, ineffective or invalidated.

Predictive value a measure that is used to interpret diagnostic tests results. This can be positive or negative.

Prevalence total number of individuals ill at any given time, and includes old and new illnesses.

Psychoprophylaxis a means of psychological conditioning that prepares women for labour through childbirth education classes during the antenatal period to enable them to utilise their own internal powers to birth their babies without the need for pharmacological methods of analgesia. This approach is popular in natural childbirth.

Puerperal psychosis an acute early onset psychiatric disorder that results in a psychiatric emergency. It is the most severe of all postpartum affective disorders.

Puerperium often referred to as the 'fourth trimester', best described as a period of recuperation following childbirth lasting for 6–8 weeks, where the uterus and other organs that underwent physiological changes in the adaptation to pregnancy, return as near as possible to their pre-pregnant state. Lactation is initiated and established, and the woman has adjusted psychologically and emotionally to the demands of motherhood.

Reciprocity simply means to give and take. It is a key component of a trusting relationship based on mutual regard and respect for the other.

Recurrence an illness returning when the individual has fully recovered.

Relapse deterioration in an individual who is already ill or not completely recovered.

Reliability in research terms this is the correlation of an item, scale or instrument with a hypothetical one that measures what it is supposed to.

Resistive behaviour onset of an acute psychotic illness such as puerperal psychosis may lead to stubborn and obstinate behaviour, where the individual refuses to comply with instructions, care and treatment, and might find it difficult to accept symptoms and diagnosis of a psychotic illness.

Risk factors adverse or vulnerability factors, hazards or variables or indeed characteristics that feature in an individual's life and put them at risk of illness. Risk factors are useful as a correlation but are not necessarily causal.

Schizophrenia a chronic, severe, and disabling psychiatric disorder with impaired brain function leading to disordered thoughts and bizarre behaviour. People with schizophrenia often experience psychosis: experience delusions and hallucinations where they may hear voices other people do not hear or may believe that others are reading their minds, controlling their thoughts, or plotting to harm them.

Secure the infant shows signs of missing the parent on departure, seeks proximity upon reunion and then returns to play. This response is associated with maternal sensitivity to infant signals and communications.

Self-concept the conscious reflection of one's self-identity i.e. how we perceive ourselves. It relates to the cognitive (thinking) aspect of the self.

Self-efficacy defined by Bandura as 'the belief in one's capabilities to organise and execute the course of action required to manage prospective situations'. In other words it is the belief a person has in their ability to achieve a goal.

Self-esteem the self-worth or opinion a person has of their value as an individual. It relates to the affective (feeling) or emotional aspect of the self.

Self-image is the mental picture, self-portrait or personal view we have of ourselves. It is the product of our learning through primary and secondary socialisation.

Self-immolation self-sacrifice e.g. setting oneself alight.

Sensitivity a statistical measure that has a positive predictive value i.e. the proportion of individuals with an illness who have a positive test result.

Specificity a statistical measure that has a negative predictive value i.e. the proportion of well individuals who have a negative test result for an illness.

Striae gravidarum stretch marks during pregnancy.

Support the social interaction between a woman and significant other – partner, relative, friend, doula or healthcare professional such as the midwife – that has a buffering effect, in that the help provided is instrumental in promoting self-determination and assisting the woman to cope in a positive manner.

Strange situation-infant-parent attachment categories   considered as the gold standard, a research procedure involving short separations from, and reunions with, the parent that assesses the quality of the attachment relationship. Based on a year-long Baltimore study of 26 infants and mothers which culminated in 60–80 hours of observation per pairing. Infant responses to this situation are categorised as: insecure-ambivalent; insecure-avoidance; insecure-disorganised/disorientated (see above).

Tokophobia   morbid fear of labour/childbirth.

Triage   defined by the Welsh Assembly Government as 'the assignment of degrees of urgency to illness or injury to decide on the order of treatment of a large number of patients'. In the maternity context where women are not usually ill, the term can be applied to an assessment area that acts as a bridge between home and labour suite. This ensures that the labour suite only receives women who are in labour or those needing to be on the labour suite for specialist care.

Validity   the extent to which a test measures what it is supposed to measure. A test needs to be valid for results to be accurately applied, interpreted and be generalisable.

'Whooley' questions   questions recommended by the National Institute for Health and Clinical Excellence (NICE) via a study by Whooley et al for use during pregnancy and post-partum periods. It is suggested that two brief focused questions that address mood and interest are as likely to be as effective as more elaborate methods for identifying depression, and are more compatible with routine use in many primary and secondary care settings.

Index

Locators shown in *italics* refer to diagrams, case vignettes, and reflective and problem-solving activities.

abnormal psychology
  as approach to understanding
    midwifery, 9
abuse, domestic
  as element of reaction to
    pregnancy, 41–2, *41–2*
acceptance (personal)
  as element of successful
    communication, 92–3, *93*
Affonso, D., 64
age, mother
  as element of reaction to
    pregnancy, 42
Ainsworth, M., 159, 163
Albany Midwifery Practice (AMP),
  150
Alexander, D., 151, 152
Alfaraj, A., 131
Altman, I., 19
AMP (Albany Midwifery Practice),
  150
Andrews, L., 158
anxiety
  as preparation for threat, 133–4
  care and management during
    pregnancy, 58–9
  during postnatal period, 66–7,
    67
  salience in childbirth, 136–9,
    137
appearances, physical
  salience in personal
    communication, 87
assertiveness
  salience in successful
    communication, 90–92, *91,
    92*
Astbury, J., 71
attachment, parent-baby
  need for by babies, 158–9
  role of cultural diversity on, 175
  see also bonding, mother-baby
attitudes, student midwife
  significance of to practice, 22–3

avoidance, cognitive
  as coping strategy, 131–2, *131,
    132*

babies
  need for bonding and
    attachment with mother,
    158–60, *159, 160*
  need for parents-baby
    attachment, 158–9
  psychosocial reactions of
    mothers to first meeting,
    160–63
  role of midwife in separation
    from parents, 165–8, *165–7*
  role of touch and tenderness in
    mother-baby communication,
    163
Balzer-Riley, J., 91, 93, 95, 96
Barlow, J., 10
Barnes, J., 163
barriers
  to effective midwife-mother
    communication, 98–9
  to successful midwife-mother
    relationships, 20–22, *21*
Bates, C., 176
Begley, C., 23
behaviourism
  as approach to understanding of
    midwifery, 2–5, *3, 4, 5*
Bem, D., 122
Bielawska-Batorowicz, E., 175
Bierhoff, H., 123, 135
biopsychology
  as approach to understanding
    midwifery, 8
bipolar disorders
  care and management during
    pregnancy, 59–61
  prevalence during perinatal
    period, 56–8, *57–8*
birth *see* childbirth
bonding, mother-baby

needs of mothers in relation to,
  159–60, *159, 160*
  see also attachment, parent baby
  see also actions enhancing e.g.
    breastfeeding; contact, skin-
    to-skin
Boscaglia, N., 31
Bradley, S., 45
brain
  salience of during process of
    childbirth, *149*
breastfeeding
  salience in maternal bonding,
    164–5
Brown, J., 57
Brownell, K., 32
Bryan, E., 44
Bryant, L., 90
bullying
  salience and impact on midwife-
    mother relationship, 22, *22*
Burke true, L., 95
Burr, V., 11
Butler, G., 128–9, 131, 133
Buunk, A., 138

Callam, R., 134
Cameron, J., 24
carers and care
  importance of type and
    continuity during pregnancy
    and childbirth, 147–51, *148,
    149*
  psychological impact of in
    relation to pregnancy and
    childbirth, 174–7
  see also examples of practice e.g.
    family-nurse partnerships;
    groups, 'pampering'; 'one-to-
    one'; Sure Start
  see also players e.g. midwives and
    midwifery; mothers
Carr, H., 31
Carver, C., 129

Chambers, M., 135
childbirth
    connection between social and
        psychological dimensions of,
        30–32, *30–31*
    emotions during, 40–46, *41–2,
        44, 46*
    evidence concerning home v.
        hospital, 103–6, *103–4*
    perceptions of pain during,
        114–17, *116*
    salience of brain during, *149*
    salience of care during, 147–51,
        148, 149, 174–6
    see also environments,
        childbirth; pregnancy
    see also influences e.g. anxiety;
        fear; midwives and midwifery
Chugani, H., 157
cognition
    as approach to understanding of
        midwifery, 5–6
Colombo, S., 45
communication
    barriers and constraints to
        effectiveness in midwife-
        mother relationships, 98–9
    humanistic approach to, 92–5,
        93–4, 95
    qualities ensuring effective,
        89–99, *92, 93,-4, 95, 96–7,
        97–8*
    psychology of, 83–7, *83–5, 86,
        88–9*
    see also relationships,
        interpersonal
    see also elements for success e.g.
        assertiveness; congruence;
        empathy; listening; presence;
        rapport
    see also specific types e.g. touch
concept, self
    definition, characteristics and
        salience of, 122
Condon, J., 159
conflict, role
    as element in transition to
        parenthood, 32–5, *33–4*
congruence
    as element of successful
        communication, 93–4,
        93–4
constraints
    on successful midwife-mother
        relationships, 20–22, *21*

to effective midwife-mother
    communication, 98–9
contact, skin-to-skin
    salience in mother-baby
        bonding, 164, *164*
control
    and coping strategies, 136
    see also power and powerlessness
Cook, R., 45
Cooper, P., 59, 67
coping
    control and, 136
    relationship with stress, 129–30,
        130
    self-efficacy and, 134–5
    strategies for, 131–2, *131, 13*
Cox, J., 54, 55, 64
culture, NHS
    impact on childbirth
        environment and experience,
        110–11, *111*

deaths, neonatal
    emotional reactions to, 44–6, *46*
de Jonge, A., 106
Deery, R., 17, 22
Dennis, C., 72
depression
    care and management during
        pregnancy, 58–9
    during perinatal period, 56–8,
        57–8
    during postnatal period, 68,
        70–72
    during puerperium, 64–7, *66, 67*
    screening tools for, 54–5, *55*
developmental psychology
    as approach to understanding
        midwifery, 8
Dick-Read, G., 115
Dijkstra, P., 138
discharge, emotional
    as coping strategy, 131–2, *131,
        132*
disorders, medical
    salience when mistaken as
        psychiatric disorders, 75–6
disorders, psychiatric
    characteristics and prevalence
        during perinatal period, 55–8,
        55–6, 57–8
    during pregnancy, 58–61
    during puerperium, 61–3, *62*
    mistaken as medical disorders,
        75–6

screening for, 53–4, 77
    see also health, maternal
        psychiatric; relationships,
        interpersonal
    see also specific diseases eg bipolar
        disorder; depression; perinatal
        mental illness
diversity, cultural
    effect on maternal attachment,
        175
Dixon, A., 18
doctors
    relationships with midwives,
        24
Donnelly, E., 83
Dornan, J., 24
doulas
    as maternal support during
        childbirth, 148
Downe, S., 105
Dykes, F., 138

Edinburgh Postnatal Depression
    Scale (EPDS), 54–5, *55*
emotions
    concerning childbirth
        environments, 106–14, *107,
        108, 110, 111–14*
    during pregnancy, childbirth
        and puerperium, 40–46, *41–2,
        44, 46*
    significance of in life, 123–7,
        123–4, 125–6
    significance of student midwife
        emotions on practice, 22–3
    see also mood
empathy
    as element of successful
        communication, 94–5, *95*
Endersby, C., 87
environments, childbirth
    advantage of home as birth
        environment, 111–14, *111–14*
    emotional, technological and
        cultural considerations
        concerning, 106–11, *107, 108,
        110*
    evidence concerning the home
        versus hospital, 103–6, *103–4*
    salience in ensuring
        psychological care of mothers,
        176–7
EPDS (Edinburgh Postnatal
    Depression Scale), 54–5, *55*
Erikson, A., 8

esteem, self
definition, characteristics and
salience of, 12
experiences, student midwife
significance of to practice,
22–3

Family Nurse Partnerships (FNPs),
46, 151
fatherhood
myths and ideologies
surrounding state of, 36–40,
37, 38, 39
role conflicts within transition
to, 32–5, *33–4*
fear
as emotional reaction to threat,
132, 133
salience in childbirth, 136–9,
137
feelings *see* emotions
feminism
as approach to understanding
midwifery, 11, *11*
Fieldman, R., 162
Florian, V., 165
FNPs (Family Nurse Partnerships),
46, 151
Folkman, S., 129–30
Foucault, M., 21–2
Freeman, L., 20
Freud, S., 2–5, *3, 4, 5* (tab)

genuineness (personal attribute)
as element of successful
communication, 93–4,
93–4
Gerhardt, S., 157
Gettler, L., 164
Glassman, W., *4*
Glover, V., 133
Goffman, E., 122
Goodall, K., 89
Grabe, S., 31
Green, J., 147
Gross, R., *4*
groups, 'pampering'
strengths as model of
care during childbirth,
151

Hadad, M., *4*
Hassin, R., 87
health, maternal psychiatric
importance, 52–3

help (concept)
psychology of giving and
receiving, 135
see *also* carers and care
Hepper, P., 157
Herbert, M., 159–60
'hierarchy of needs' (Maslow),
6–8
Hildebrand, J., 20
Hodnett, E., 107
home
advantages of as childbirth
environment, 111–14, *111–14*
evidence concerning home v.
hospital as childbirth
environment, 103–6, *103–4*
Hope, T., 128–9, 131, 133
hormones
influence of during childbirth,
115–17, *116, 149*
hospitals
evidence concerning hospital v.
home as childbirth
environment, 103–6, *103–4*
Huang, L., 43
humanism
as approach to understanding
communication, 92–5, *93–4,
95*
as approach to understanding
midwifery, 6–8, *6, 7*
Hunter, B., 17, 20, 22, 106–7
Hyde, L., 31

'ideal self'
role in self-regulation, 127–8,
127
illness *see* disorders
image, body
relevance to psychological
health, 30–33, *30–31, 33*
see *also influences on e.g.* media
impressions, human
psychology of first impressions,
86–7, *86*
inconsistency
defending the self from,
128–9
intrauterine fetal death (IUD),
44–6, *46*

Johnson, M., 138

Kaufmann, T., 12
Kirkham, M., 17, 18, 20, 107

knowledge, self
salience of creating consistency
of, 122–8, *123–4, 125–6,
127*
Kumar, R., 64

labour *see* childbirth
Lazarus, R., 128, 129–30
Lewis, G., 41
limbic system
definition, characteristics and
salience, 125–7, *125–6*
listening
as element of successful
midwife-mother
communication, 95–8, *96–7,
97–8*
Lorberbaum, J., 163

MacArthur, C., 152
McKenna, J., 164
Mackie, D., 86, 124, 129
McKinlay, A., 8–9, 12
MacLachlan, M., 11, 175
McVittie, A., 8–9, 12
Maio, G., 32
managed-care networks, 74
Markowic, D., 20
Marris, P., 139
Maslow, A., 6–8
Mearns, D., 90, 97
media
psychological influence on body
image, 31–2
medicalisation
of childbirth environment,
109–10, *110*
see *also influences determining eg*
attitudes, midwife; homes;
hospitals
Mehrabian, A., 86
midwives and midwifery
impact of fear, anxiety and stress
on, 132–4, 136–9, *137*, 174–6
relationship with doctors, 24
role and salience as key figure in
maternal support, 38–40, *39*,
147–8, 152
role in cases of perinatal mental
illness, 72–4, *73*
salience of feminism to
understanding of, 11, *11*
see *also* babies; childbirth;
mothers; pregnancies and
pregnancy; students, midwife

see also concerns and influences
  e.g. coping; emotions;
  psychology; stress
see also elements of e.g.
  communication; rapport,
  reciprocity; relationships,
  interpersonal
Mikulincer, M., 165
Miller, G., 132
mind, fetal
  development of in preparation
    for interpersonal
    relationships, 157–8
miscarriage
  emotional reactions to, 44–6,
    46
models and theories
  history and relevance of
    psychological, 2–12, *3, 4, 5, 6,*
    7, 8, 9, 10–11, 12
  of care practice during
    childbirth, 150–51
  see also name e.g. behaviourism;
    biopsychology; cognition;
    hierarchy of needs;
    humanism; psychoanalysis
Moller, K., 176
mood
  disorders during perinatal
    period, 55–6, *55–6*
  disorders during puerperium,
    61–3, *62*
  during postpartum period,
    68–70, 68–9
mothers and motherhood
  actors and situations ensuring
    successful care of, 176–7
  impact of cultural diversity on
    attachment with baby, 175
  importance of continuity and
    type of carer, 147–51, *148,*
    149
  myths and ideologies
    surrounding state of, 35–6, *35,*
    36
  psychosocial reactions on seeing
    babies for first time, 160–63
  role conflicts within transition
    to, 32–5, *33–4*
  role in baby attachment and
    bonding, 158–60, *159,*
    160
  role of touch and tenderness in
    mother-baby communication,
    163

see also age, mother; midwives
  and midwifery; parents and
  parenthood; relationships,
  interpersonal
see also elements of relationships
  e.g. communication; rapport
see also help required e.g. support,
  psychosocial
"mothering the mother"
  as element of midwife-mother
  relationship, 20
Murray, L., 55–6, 59, 67,
  158

National Health Service
  impact of organisation of on
  childbirth environment
  and experience, 110–11,
  111
Nelson-Jones, R., 93, 97
Neville, L., 83
Nicholson, P., 68

Oates, M., 9, 65, 75
obesity versus thinness
  psychological impact on body
  image, 32, *33*
obsessive-compulsive disorders
  during postnatal period, 66–7,
  67
O'Connor, T., 133
Odent, M., 116–17
Ogden, J., 9–10, 11, 129, 132
O'Hara, M., 55–6, 57
Oliver, R., 87
'one-to-one'
  strengths as model of care
  during childbirth, 150
O'Reilly, A., 35–6
organisation, NHS
  impact on childbirth
  environment and experience,
  110–11, *111*
'ought self'
  role in self-regulation, 127–8,
  127

Page, L., 18, 106, 147, 150
pain
  psychological perceptions of in
  childbirth, 114–17, *116*
Pandora, A., 134
parents and parenthood
  role conflicts within transition
  to, 32–5, *33–4*

role of midwife in separation of
  parents from baby, 165–8,
  165–7
see also attachment, parent-
  baby; mothers and
  motherhood
Parkinson, P., 88
partners
  as key figure in maternal support
  during childbirth, 148
partnerships
  family nurse, 46, 151
Pembroke, J., 19–20
Pembroke, M., 19–20
perinatal mental illness
  characteristics and description,
  51–2
  role of midwives in cases of,
  72–4, *73*
  see also health, maternal
  psychiatric
Perry, C., 151, 152
Phoenix, A., 68
peurperium, the
  connection between social and
  psychological dimensions of,
  30–32, *30–31*
  emotions during, 40–46, *41–2,*
  44, 46
  mood disorders during, 621–3,
  622
  normative adjustment reactions
  during, 44–6, *46*
Pinel, J., 8
Plantin, L., 38–9
PMI *see* perinatal mental illness
postpartum
  care and management of
  psychiatric disorders during,
  61–3, *62*
  incidence, aetiology and
  management of depression
  during, 64–7, *66, 67*
  incidence, aetiology and
  management of mood
  disorders during, 68–70,
  68–9
  significance of suicide during,
  74–5
power and powerlessness
  as element of childbirth
  environment, 107
  in midwife-mother relationship,
  20–22, *21*
  see also control

pregnancies and pregnancy
  connection between social and
    psychological dimensions of,
    30–32, *30–31*
  emotions during, 40–46, *41–2,*
    44, 46
  importance of care during,
    147–9, *148, 149*
  normative adjustment
    reactions, 40–43, *41–2*
  psychiatric disorders during,
    58–61
  significance of suicide during,
    74–5
  see also players involved e.g.
    midwives and midwifery;
    mothers and motherhood;
    partners
presence (personal attribute)
  as element of successful
    communication, 96–8, *96–7.,*
    97–8
presentation, self (personal
    attribute)
  definition, characteristics and
    salience, 128
psychoanalysis
  as approach to understanding of
    midwifery, 2
psychology
  during pregnancy, childbirth
    and peurperium, 30–32,
    30–31, 174–6
  history, potential and relevance
    to midwifery, 2–12, *3, 4, 5, 6,*
    7, 8, 9, 10–11, 12, 173–4, *173,*
    174
  of childbirth environment,
    176–8
  of childbirth pain perceptions,
    114–17, *116*
  of communication, 83–7, *83–5,*
    86, 88–9
  see also e.g. coping; power and
    powerlessness; rapport
  see also situations influenced
    eg environments,
    childbirth; relationships,
    interpersonal
psychosis
  care and management of during
    puerperium, 63–4
  incidence, aetiology and
    features of during
    puerperium, 61–3, *62*

puerperium
  emotions during, 40–46, *41–2,*
    44, 46
  incidence, aetiology and
    features of psychiatric
    disorders during, 61–4, *62*
  incidence, aetiology and
    management of depression
    during, 64–7, *66, 67*

Raphael-Leff, J., 136, 160
rapport
  role in midwife-mother
    communication, 85–6, *85–6*
Raskin, N., 93
Raynor, M., 9, 34
reactions, psychosocial
  of mothers to seeing baby for
    first time, 160–63
reciprocity
  as element of midwife-mother
    relationship, 19
Redshaw, M., 43
relationships, interpersonal
  development of and the fetal
    mind, 157–8
  emotional and psychological
    considerations, 106–14, *107,*
    108, 110, 111–14
  midwife-doctor, 24
  midwife-mother, 16–22, *17–18,*
    21, 22
  psychology of building between
    midwife and mother, 88–9,
    88, 89
  significance and frequency of,
    90
  see also influences e.g.
    communication
responses, physical
  salience in communication, 87
risk
  during perinatal period, 55–6,
    55–6
  during postnatal period, 68, 71
  during puerperium, 61–3, *62*
  see also safety
Robertson, E., 61
Robling, S., 67
Rodriguez, C., 131
Rogers, C., 6–7, 92, 94, 95
Rotter, J., 136
Rowe, D., 131
rumination
  as coping strategy, 131

safety
  as element of midwife-mother
    relationship, 18
  see also risk
Satir, V., 98
Schafer, W., 98
schemas, self, 123
Scheri, F., 164
schizophrenia
  care and management during
    pregnancy, 59–61
  during perinatal period, 56–8,
    57–8
Schott, J., 90, 96
Schwartz, M., 32
screening
  for psychiatric disorders, 53–4,
    77
  see also tools, screening
Segerstrom, S., 132
self image, body
  relevance to psychological
    health, 30–33, *30–31, 33*
  see also influences on e.g. media
separation, parent-baby
  role of midwife in, 165–8, *165–7*
Shahidullah, P., 157
Shipley, J., 31
Siddiqui, A., 175
Siddiqui, J., 15, 23
Simkin, P., 115
Simon, B., 123
Skouteris, H., 31
Smith, A., 18
Smith, E., 86, 124, 129
social constructivism
  as approach to understanding
    midwifery, 11–12
social psychology
  as approach to understanding
    midwifery, 8–9, *9*
socialisation, student midwife
  significance of to practice, 22–3
spirituality
  as element of midwife-mother
    relationship, 19–20
Stapleton, H., 107
Stern, A., 157–8
strategies, coping *see* coping
stress
  defending the self from, 128–9
  impact on midwives of, 138–9,
    175–6
  relationship with coping
    strategies, 129–30, *130*

Stuart, S., 132, 133
students, midwife
    significance of attitudes,
        experiences and emotions to
        practice, 22–3
suicide
    significance in pregnancy and
        postpartum period, 74–5
support, psychosocial
    definition in characteristics,
        144–5, *144, 145*
    evidential assessment of levels
        an extent, 145–7, *146*
    see also key players e.g. midwives
        and midwifery; partners
    see also examples of e.g. groups,
        'pampering'; visits, listening
Sure Start
    strengths as model of care
        during childbirth, 151
Swain, A., 55–6, 57
Swain, J., 161, 162, 163

Taylor, D., 19
Taylor, J., 24
technology, use of
    psychological impact on
        childbirth environment
        relationships, 107–8, *108*
tenderness
    role in mother-baby
        communication, 163

theories and models *see* models
    and theories
'theory of consciousness' (Freud),
    2–5, *3, 4, 5*
thinness versus obesity
    psychological impact on body
        image, 32, *33*
Thompson, F., 23
Thorne, P., 97
togetherness (personal
    attribute)
    needs of mothers in relation to
        mother-baby togetherness,
        159–60, *159, 160*
tools, screening
    antenatal psychiatric disorders,
        77
    for psychiatric disorders, 54–6,
        55–6
Torner, L., 161
touch
    as element of successful
        midwife-mother
        communication, 96–8, *96–7,*
        97–8
    role in mother-baby
        communication, 163
Trope, Y., 87
Trötschel, R., 123
trust
    as element of midwife-mother
        relationship, 19

unconditional positive regard
    as element of successful
        communication, 92–3,
        93

Van Teijlingen, E., 109–110
violence
    and impact on midwife-mother
        relationship, 22, *22*
visits, listening
    strengths as model of care
        during childbirth, 151

Walsh, D., 20, 105
Ward, S., 31
Watt, M., 132, 133
warmth
    as element of successful
        communication, 92–3,
        93
Wertheim, E., 31
White, O., 175
Whooley questions, 54, *55*
Wiggins, M., 151
Wilkinson, R., 164
Williams, C., 135
Winnicott, D., 161, 163
Woollett, A., 68
Workmeister, G., 104
Wright, B., 83

Yearsley, C., 23

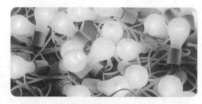
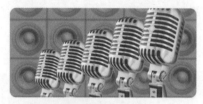
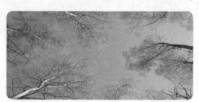
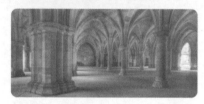
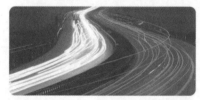
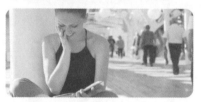
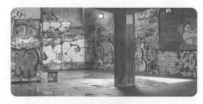